MAIN LIBRARY

OVERSIZE

ACPL ITEM
DISCARDED

S0-EBV-404

646.726 Sch6L   7086306
Schorr, Lia.
Lia Schorr's Skin care guide
for men

DO NOT REMOVE
CARDS FROM POCKET

ALLEN COUNTY PUBLIC LIBRARY

FORT WAYNE, INDIANA 46802

You may return this book to any agency, branch,
or bookmobile of the Allen County Public Library.

DEMCO

"Every man looks better once he knows Lia Schorr. Lia's got the touch—she can convince a man that his skin is worth saving, and she can show him exactly how to go about it in the easiest, most effective way."

—Camille Duhé
Grooming Editor
Gentlemen's Quarterly

"The woman who helps men put their best face forward is undoubtedly Lia Schorr! Her intelligent, easy-to-follow advice for skin care works all the time."

—Lynne Carol Dorsey
Entertainment Editor
Us magazine

"I thoroughly enjoyed my facial at the Lia Schorr Skin Care Salon. My skin felt refreshed and I was amazed at how relaxed I felt after her treatment. I honestly thought I'd never looked better. Her treatments aren't just a lifestyle of the rich and famous—they're a necessity for everybody!"

—Robin Leach
Lifestyles of the Rich and Famous

"Lia Schorr's pioneering effort to bring sound skin care advice to men has made her one of the few skin care experts to earn the praise and cooperation of dermatologists—as well as making her a sought-after authority in this field. Ms. Schorr's skin programs are truly therapeutic. This book is an important first step for any man who is truly interested in his appearance."

—John F. Romano, M.D.
NYC Dermatologist

"Now at last a book for men on how to take care of our skin. Lia Schorr's SKIN CARE GUIDE FOR MEN is packed full of the marvelous easy to follow information and helpful tips that have made her "For Men Only" skin care course such a hit at The Learning Annex."

—Bill Zanker
President
The Learning Annex

"Athletes suffer more wear and tear on their skin than the average person. They are constantly exposed to the damaging, cumulative effects of the sun's ultraviolet rays, and the residue left on the skin from the dust and perspiration after a good workout can cause blemishes. Every athlete should learn to take care of his (or her) skin from the earliest possible age, and there's no better teacher than Lia Schorr."

—Kim Cunningham
Senior Editor
World Tennis

"Lia Schorr has long known the importance of good nutrition to healthy, attractive skin—and she knows how to recognize clues to poor eating habits in her clients' appearance. I value her insights into the important field of skin care—and trust that her book will make an important contribution to a man's looks and self-awareness."

—Samuel S. Bursuk, M.D.
Consulting Health Educator
Nutritionist

"Lia has been working with me for a few years, and I can certainly tell you how pleased I am with her treatment and handling of my face. I support her system wholeheartedly."

—Shepherd Brandfon
Vice-President, Publisher
1001 Home Ideas

"In the overly hyped, pretentious world of skin care writing, Lia Schorr is a breath of fresh air. As a regular feature writer in **Better Nutrition** and **Today's Living** magazines, she has become one of our most popular contributors. Her no-nonsense, down-to-earth tips about skin care are both refreshing and enlightening. If a certain ingredient or approach doesn't work, she tells you so. Of special interest to our readers are her practical suggestions about nutrition and how numerous environmental agents may affect the skin. We have learned to respect her recommendations."

—Frank Murray
Associate Publisher/Editor
Better Nutrition and **Today's Living**

"Because I travel a lot my skin takes a beating. I never considered going for professional skin care until a good friend of mine suggested it. Now I'm hooked—Lia's program has helped my skin look and feel a lot better than I ever expected."

—John Dominis
Photographer

"Besides being a dedicated professional, Lia Schorr is a recognized expert in the field of skin care. She was one of the very first to realize that this is an issue of concern to men as well as to women. Because I'm concerned with giving the readers of my magazine, **Muscle & Fitness,** only the most authoritative and up-to-date information, I picked Lia to write our monthly skin care column. Because I believe in her advice, I follow it myself."

—Joe Weider
Publisher, **Muscle & Fitness**
Trainer of Champions Since 1936

Lia Schorr's

SKIN CARE
GUIDE
FOR MEN

LIA SCHORR'S

SKIN CARE GUIDE FOR MEN

Lia Schorr
With Shari Miller

Prentice-Hall, Inc.   Englewood Cliffs, N.J.

Prentice-Hall International, Inc., **London**
Prentice-Hall of Australia, Pty. Ltd., **Sydney**
Prentice-Hall Canada Inc., **Toronto**
Prentice-Hall of India Private Ltd., **New Delhi**
Prentice-Hall of Japan, Inc., **Tokyo**
Prentice-Hall of Southeast Asia Pte. Ltd., **Singapore**
Whitehall Books, Ltd., **Wellington, New Zealand**
Editora Prentice-Hall do Brasil Ltda., **Rio de Janeiro**
Prentice-Hall Hispanoamericana, S.A., **Mexico**

Allen County Public Library
Ft. Wayne, Indiana

© 1985 by
Lia Schorr

All rights reserved. No part of this
book may be reproduced in any form or
by any means, without permission in
writing from the publisher.

This book is a reference work based on research by
the author. The opinions expressed herein are not
necessarily those of or endorsed by the publisher.
The directions stated in this book are in no way to
be considered as a substitute for consultation with
a duly licensed doctor.

Library of Congress Cataloging in Publication Data

Schorr, Lia.
Lia Schorr's skin care guide for men.

Includes index.
1. Skin—Care and hygiene. 2. Men—Health and
hygiene. 3. Grooming for men. I. Miller, Shari.
II. Title. III. Title: Skin care guide for men.
RL87.S346 1985   646.7'26   85-3501
ISBN 0-13-535121-9
ISBN 0-13-535113-8 (PBK)

Printed in the United States of America

ABOUT LIA SCHORR

7086306

When you ask one of Lia's clients to describe her, they use adjectives like "energetic" … "talented" … "knowledgeable" … "inspiring." They tell you that "she makes skin care simple" … "she doesn't go in for puffery or miracle claims" … that "she is logical and intelligent." Perhaps that is why, in the almost 20 years she has been in the skin care business, so many men—some of them famous, and many of them not-so-famous—have put their skin in her hands.

Lia Schorr prides herself in helping to raise men's skin care awareness, in sharing her expertise with men from every walk of life, of every age, in every career. In the seven years she worked at the Georgette Klinger salon in New York City, she helped establish their men's salon and make it the success it later became. When she founded her own salon in May of 1980, she formulated a line of skin care products specifically for men—and found her male clientele soon increasing from 30 percent to the 60 percent it is today. The source of her special rapport with men, say many of her male clients, is that she treats them with intelligence and gives them skin care **facts,** not myths.

Lia was born in Russia to Polish parents who had immigrated there to escape from the Nazis. She lived briefly in Poland, after which her parents moved the family to Israel in 1950. Lia's interest in skin care began while living in a kibbutz and serving in the Israeli army—both environments in which discipline and pride in oneself were encouraged. She received her formal skin care training in France, then came to New York City, where she has practiced skin care since.

Lia's important contributions to the skin care field have been noted widely around the world. Lia has appeared on television on **The Today Show, Cable Health Network, P.M. Magazine, Two On The Town, A.M. Chicago, Channel 4 News** (NYC), **Channel 7 News** (NYC), and **Saturday Morning Live,** discussing men's skin care and giving hard-hitting advice. She has been interviewed on 40 radio shows across the country and has been a steady guest on **WMCA** radio in New York City, answering questions on the topic of men's skin care.

Lia's skin care tips have appeared in countless magazines in the U.S., Europe, Israel, and South America, including **GQ, Esquire, Town & Country, Travel & Leisure, Vogue,** and **Harper's Bazaar.** Lia has also been featured in **People** magazine and **Us.** In addition, she writes skin care columns for a variety of magazines including **Fit, Shape, Muscle & Fitness,** and **Better Nutrition.** She has also been featured in newspapers across the country as well as in the **New York Post.**

v

For the past three years, Lia has taught a skin care class exclusively for men at **The Learning Annex** in New York City. She is a member of the Society of Cosmetic Chemists, Cosmetic Executive Women, and The Fashion Group.

In addition to treating clients in her salon, Lia has an extensive—and growing—mail order business.

SHARI MILLER is a beauty and fitness writer for a major fashion magazine. Based in New York City, her work has appeared in a variety of national magazines as well as in newspapers.

Dedicated to all men of sensitivity
who take pride in themselves ...
and to my daughter, Segaal, who
has brought magic and pleasure
into my life.

CONTENTS

ACKNOWLEDGMENTS

First of all, I thank my editor, Bette Schwartzberg, for believing in me and helping to make my dream of a book a reality. I also thank Shari Miller, the writer who devoted her time, her talent, and her friendship to this project. Susan Wides—the photographer whose work is seen later in these pages—and the illustrator Lamont O'Neal—also deserve appreciation for their understanding and the quality of their work, as do all the men who so graciously allowed us to photograph them for use in my book.

I also thank everyone who stood behind me during the past four years since I opened my own business—friends, family, clients, and especially members of the press, who helped me to bring needed information on men's skin care to a wider audience. All of these special people helped me to build my skin care salon and loyal clientele faster than I had ever hoped.

Lia Schorr

INTRODUCTION

Why a skin care book for men, you ask?

Because I have yet to meet a man who doesn't care about how he looks. And as women have known for years, skin is where it all begins.

Every time I am interviewed on men's skin care in **Esquire** or **GQ** magazines, the floodgates open. So many letters and calls come in, I barely have time to answer them all. "Where can I get that product?" they want to know. "Can you do anything to remove these scars?" "How can I stop my face from breaking out?" Or simply, "When can I schedule a facial?" Like the woman in the TV commercial, men are finally beginning to say, "I'm worth it."

Until now, men had nowhere to go for hard-hitting skin care advice. They were afraid of being seen as vain, effeminate, or ignorant if they stepped into a skin care salon. Marching up to a counter in a department store seemed equally embarassing. So, they sneaked products from their wives' or girlfriends' side of the medicine cabinet, and tried a little of this plus a little of that (I've heard this confession at least once a day). Maybe they snuck a look at a woman's magazine—if a particular skin care column (**Cooling that sunburn...**say) caught their eye. Maybe they just thought that time would clear the problem up—and, unfortunately, in the skin care business, time is nobody's friend.

Right now the major cosmetics companies are pouring millions of dollars into the creation of skin care products for men—products that men haven't the faintest idea how to **use.** Most men can handily rattle off vital statistics like their height, their weight, how much "iron" they can pump, and their favorite baseball player's batting average, but they have no idea whether their skin—the largest and most visible human organ—is dry, oily, or in-between. This lack of knowledge wouldn't be so bad if it didn't lead to needless rashes, allergies, blemishes, irritations, and even permanent scars. When these occur, men blame the Hand of Fate, the mood they're in, or the products they're using, rather than themselves. Their own lack of knowledge, simply put, is their skin's worst enemy.

Perhaps you're one of those men who think that simply because you're a man, your skin should be taking care of itself. All those lotions and potions, you think, are just for women. Maybe, once upon a time, when we lived in a pollutant-free, stress-free, weather-free world, your skin could get by on its own. Nowadays the world isn't cooperating. And that's why I believe **men need a skin care book for themselves.**

What you'll find in the following chapters is a systematic guide to preventing the most serious skin problems men face. From acne scarring to premature aging to the daily cross men have to bear—shaving irritation.

This book deals with problems specific to men, like shaving, hormone cycles, hair growth—or the lack of it. It includes, in every chapter, plenty of do-it-yourself advice for those men still too shy to get themselves to a skin care salon. Most importantly, it is easy enough for every man to follow. My philosophy is that the sooner you learn good skin care habits, the better. There's no reason for skin care to be complicated—and the advice in this book isn't.

In fact, this book will be the only skin care book a man will ever need. Nearly every time I give a man his first facial, he says, "Now why didn't I ever think of this before?" To me, "before" doesn't really matter. What matters is that he—and all the readers of this book—finally cares enough about himself to think about his skin **now.**

CHAPTER ONE

WHY I WROTE THIS BOOK—
AND WHY EVERY MAN SHOULD READ IT

I never met a man I didn't like.

—Will Rogers

I care about the way you look because **you care.** Sixty percent of the clients in my New York City salon are men—some of them barely old enough to shave, some in the prime of their lives, some in their twenties, some in their eighties. They all have one thing in common: They want to look their best.

You're no exception. That's why you're reading this book. Think about the amount of time you spend at your gym or health club. Think about the amount of money you donated this year to your hair stylist or your tailor or even your dentist. Think about what you sucked in, or puffed out, the last time you looked in a mirror. Imagine the last time someone complemented you on your appearance. If it hasn't happened lately, why not? And if it has, then admit it, you ate it up.

I'm not a psychic, but when a man comes into my office for any reason, I know a lot about him **instantly.** I know whether he gets enough exercise—or considers walking back and forth between the refrigerator and the TV set a nightly workout. I know whether he's been spending too many lunch hours living out of a donut box. I know if he's been abusing alcohol or drugs. I can tell whether his life is full of happiness or stress. It's all written on his skin.

Bare skin doesn't lie, and my heart goes out to you men whenever something misfires or erupts or generally interferes with your skin's natural balance. **You can't cover it with makeup,** the way a woman can.

Your skin is the largest organ in your body. You may treat it as if it's made of armor, but it's actually just as vulnerable as lace, and it takes a pummeling from morning till night. A man's skin isn't all that different from a woman's skin—just somewhat rougher on the outside—but it gets treated a whole lot differently.

I've been in the skin care business for almost 20 years, and I have yet to meet a man whose skin didn't need some kind of special care. In fact, the biggest skin problem I see is between the ears, in the mind. It's a question of

attitude. You may have the mistaken belief that just because you're a man, your skin should need less care than a woman's. You have a hard time imagining, say, a famous movie star lying still for a facial, or a big-name Wall Street broker doing the same. But I know for a fact they do, in my salon.

Actually, your skin is biologically programmed to bounce back from a great deal of very inelegant tortures. If you have a photograph of your great-great grandfather—perhaps leaning against a sod hut in the great American outdoors—he probably had "perfect" skin (assuming he'd escaped smallpox and the rigors of nonelectric shaving). He also ate preservative-free foods, drank cleaner water than you'll ever know, and worked out by felling a row of maples before breakfast.

His son took on all the problems of industrialized society. **His** son took on all those problems in double-time. Now there's you. You've got a similar genetic code to your grandfather, but you've also got that many more skin enemies of your own. You've got everything to learn about defending your skin against the hazards of modern life.

Recently I had a typical visit from a man in my salon. He entered my office with his wife and mother-in-law. He had some acne scarring and was interested in my advice as to what could be done to lessen it. He was an intelligent, articulate man, a success in his career, but he hardly said a word for ten minutes.

"What can you do about his scars?" asked the wife.

"What kind of skin does he have?" asked the mother-in-law.

"Can he treat his skin at home?" asked the wife.

"What about deep-peeling treatments?" asked the mother-in-law.

I'm not for a moment implying that this man was shy or henpecked or stupid. It's just that men don't have the vocabulary to approach skin care. With women, skin terminology is as natural as breathing. I believe that, with time, men will come to know just as much.

I know the interest is there. Every day I receive letters from men in all walks of life—athletes, students, politicians, artists, servicemen, retirees. They have all sorts of questions that aren't being answered by any book that I have come across—and believe me, I've looked. The questions are very often the same, very often about "insignificant" problems—a pimple here and there, a rash, ingrown hairs, oily skin. But they are significant problems when they're **your** problem.

Maybe you've gotten this far in life and your skin is still perfect (although I've yet to meet anyone who thought this about their own skin). Or at least you don't have problems serious enough to warrant "special" treatments. But that's **now.** You've been lucky. Your skin will not stay the same. Its chemistry will change. You may go through a period of stress that will wreak havoc on your spirits—and your skin. You may overdo the sun— and you never do realize the damage the sun does until it's already too late.

Good skin care is like preventive medicine. It teaches you what to do now to avoid undesirable effects later. I can teach you how to treat skin that's acting up (gently), how to pep up tired skin, even how to avoid speeding up the natural aging process, although no one can yet teach us how to slow it down. In other words, I can help you to prevent problems in your skin as time goes on.

And I am interested in something else: pampering. We live in one of those rare civilizations in which men have learned absolutely nothing about pampering themselves. Sure, your mother pampered you when you were a baby, and somewhere deep down you remember what that feels like. You deserve to have that feeling **now**—and to learn how to give it to yourself. Most of life's best sensations pass through your skin—but how much real attention do you ever pay **it**?

Before I talk about what you should be doing, I'll address what you're probably doing now....

Is your day something like this? You wake up in the morning and shower with whatever soap you happen to find in the tub today. You run a razor across your face. The razor burns a bit (you're in a hurry as usual), so you splash on some aftershave. It burns even more. You're out the door. Your skin begins to react to the season—if it's winter, your face (the most exposed part of your body, in every weather) starts to redden. If it's summer, and you're in any kind of rush, you will probably start to perspire. In fact, by the time you've arrived at your office, you've probably already worked up a healthy sweat.

You may have also done quite a bit to alter your body—and your skin—chemistry. It may be barely 10 A.M., but a lot's been going on. You've poured yourself a cup of coffee, maybe even lit up a cigarette. You then begin to work full-out all day. **Still** more chemicals (any kind of stress, good **or** bad, has a chemical effect on the body). After work, maybe you stop by the health club to work out all the tension you've built up during the day.

During that time, have you paid **any** attention to your skin? It's done a pretty good job of taking care of you, of sealing out the environment, but let's take a look at all the ways you've abused **it**.

First of all, the shower. If you were using soap, did you take a look at the ingredients in that particular brand? Do you have any idea of what's actually **in** soap? Most soap manufacturers make a product that's powerful enough to remove a week's worth of grime from under the dirtiest construction worker's fingernails. This is fine, especially if your hands are dirty. But do you really need all that power on your **face**? Just like women, men have sensitive skin. How many times have you found your skin reacting badly to a particular product and just continued using it—never suspecting that it may be the soap's fault rather than your skin's. How many times would you let your car bump or grind or smoke without taking it in for a checkup? You wouldn't consider still driving it, would you? Then why keep abusing your skin when it is obviously reacting to something unfavorably? I recommend that my clients not use soap at all, but more on that later.

Now let's talk about shaving. Here you are taking a sharpened piece of metal and running it across one of the most sensitive parts of your body. Sometimes you even draw blood—the necessary price you have to pay to be presentable? Not at all. You probably learned to shave from your harried, not-so-terribly-informed father, who in turn learned from **his** father. Your father and grandfather were not skin care specialists. Chances are their skin was not even exactly the same as yours. They taught you bad or misinformed habits that you repeat almost every day of your life. You walk around with needless cuts, even needless rashes. I've had clients who absolutely hated shaving—until I taught them the better way. I taught them, among other things, that applying a burning aftershave is **not** the right way to care for your skin. Burning skin that's already been traumatized by shaving is like applying salt to an open wound. I've taught them the proper way to prepare a beard, the proper way to shave, the proper care of the skin **after** shaving—and I'll teach you, too, later in this book.

Now let's take your exit out into the elements. Let's say it's December, a howling blizzard, and by the time you get to the bus stop or train station, your face is numb and red. Have you taken any precautions to protect your face from this onslaught of wind and cold? If you could see yourself now, you'd probably observe that your body's natural protection system has gone to work—the blood vessels in your face are working overtime, accounting for the redness you see. If you don't have a beard or aren't wearing a ski mask, you're probably asking a bit too much of your face. You wouldn't go out into a blizzard barefoot, yet the skin of your face is many times less durable than the soles of your feet. The effects of overexposure start to add up, and eventually what you'll get is chapped, flaking skin. Yet this doesn't have to be the course that your skin takes. If you'll read on, I can tell you simple ways to keep this from happening.

Now take a summer day, the day you work up a sweat just getting from your front door to your desk or spot in a factory. What's wrong with a little sweat, you ask, it's natural, right? Well, the bacteria on your skin agree, they just love it when you sweat. They love to multiply on your back and your chest and your neck—especially the area under your shirt collar that never seems to get any air. Lo and behold, the bacteria also multiply on your face. Before you know it, your skin starts to break out. Maybe just a little bit, or maybe a lot. But most men feel that even **one** pimple is one too many. And you'll certainly feel that way once you realize that breakouts do not have to happen, that the majority of them can be prevented.

Now let's talk about your day at work. Take all the cumulative effects of stress, caffeine, cigarettes...and what about what you had—or didn't have—

for lunch? What did you drink during a typical workday? If you're like many men, you probably relaxed by having at least one drink by the end of the day, either at lunch or at a favorite neighborhood hangout. Rather than alcohol, what your skin needs is **water**. Instead of "relaxing" with a drink, you might be better off trying exercise or having a facial. That's right. A facial. Women relax in salons all the time—even the new breed of executive women—so why shouldn't you?

Maybe you think that exercise can take care of everything, work off all your excesses of food and drink and stress, that an hour of virtue can make up for a life of "vice." Well, exercise is a **start**, but it's not all there is to health or well-being.

You need—and deserve—more. Like it or not, your face is a road map of the life you've lived up to now. To understand the connection between the inside and the outside of you, you need to understand how your skin works. You need to know what type of skin you have, so you'll know what kinds of products to buy for yourself (yes, I'll teach you how to be so smart that you won't have to steal the wrong moisturizers from your wife's or lover's side of the cabinet). You need to understand the difference between inevitable aging and sun-induced aging—and to know the difference that the right diet and the right exercise plan can make in your health and your appearance. I'm not asking for lots of time spent on your skin—no more than you're spending right now. You don't even have to spend a lot of money. But you owe it to yourself to spend the time and money you're spending right now correctly, for your own benefit, not for anyone else's.

You may have noticed that bookstores are full of skin care books for women. Maybe parts of those books could apply to you. But you need a book **just for you.** Your skin **is** different from a woman's. Shaving has toughened it. Your hormones are different. You age differently.

Most of all, though, I hope this book will change your attitude, even just a little. I'll be the first to admit that many men are skeptical when they come to me for a facial for the first time—or come to one of my lectures in New York. But they leave convinced. The most gratifying thing for me to hear is a man saying, "If I had known it would be like this, I would have been here a long time ago."

This book will show you how to take your skin through the course of a day. Through the course of the seasons. Through the course of your life. This book is for men with problem skin and men with perfect skin. This book is for teenagers and men just starting to notice the aging process. This book is for men whose faces are their living and for men who just want to look that extra bit better. This book is for all men.

CHAPTER TWO

LEARNING ABOUT YOUR SKIN

Health and intellect are the two blessings of life.

—Menander

American men spend over $20 million yearly on skin care products, according to industry analysts. Yet ask the typical American male what type of skin he has—what his basis for **choosing** a skin care product should be—and he is likely to say something like, "I think my skin is a little dry," or, "I guess my skin is oily; I used to break out when I was in my teens." If this man's age is 40, his answer shows that he really hasn't been paying as much attention to his skin as he may think. In this chapter, I'll show you how to be certain of what your skin's natural tendencies are, how your skin works, and how and why the needs of your skin may actually change with the changing seasons.

YOUR SKIN TYPE: WHERE SKIN CARE BEGINS

Whether your skin is dry, oily, or a combination of the two (as most men's skin tends to be) depends on many factors. Your skin is living, changing tissue. It is affected by heredity (more on this later); by aging; by the state of your health; by the environment you live in, indoors and outside; by the ratio of stress and relaxation in your life; and by the type and amount of food, alcohol, and medication you take in. Just as few men live by the exact same routine month in and month out, your skin also can shift in its needs from one season to the next, one year to another. Just as you are probably not wearing all the same clothes this month as you did a few months or years ago, you may not be correct in thinking you can use the same skin care products throughout every month of the year.

A man must also be aware that shaving, which most men do on a daily or every-other-day basis, can radically affect the nature of your skin. (For this reason, I've devoted an entire chapter to the how to's and how not to's of a perfect shave.) In using the advice I'll be giving you now, be aware that it pertains primarily to the area of your face where you **don't** shave, i.e., from the cheeks to the hairline. This is your most "natural" skin, your most unprotected skin, and the skin too many men ignore. The best way to determine your skin type is to have it analyzed by a professional skin care expert. But with the following hints, you can do the next-best thing: Analyze your skin under an expert's guidance.

The Cotton-Ball Test

First use this highly-visual, simple test to get a general idea of your skin type. To begin, mix up the following tonic: In a blender, combine the juice of one lemon, ½ cup of distilled water, 1 teaspoon of olive oil and three ice cubes. Blend till the ice is melted. Then brush your hair off your face and cleanse your skin, using a gentle cleansing lotion rather than soap. Finish by recleansing the skin using cotton balls wet with the tonic. Wait three hours. Wet three clean cotton balls with the tonic. Using a circular motion, gently wipe the first cotton ball across your forehead, the second down your nose, the third across one cheek. If all three come up clean your skin is probably dry; if they're dark, it's oily; if they're slightly soiled, your skin, like most men's, is a combination of the two.

Now that you have a general idea of your skin type, it's time to take a closer look at your skin. Choose a room that is brightly lit (near a window in daylight is ideal; flourescent light will be least flattering), and have a magnifying mirror handy.

- **Look at your skin's surface.** Are there uneven, flaky patches that seem to lift up from the surface? Do you see any red areas or parched-looking areas? These are further signs of dry skin.

- **Examine your nose.** Does it often look shiny within a few hours of cleansing? Do you see tiny blackheads, whiteheads, or skin eruptions? (More on these in the next chapter.) If so, your skin in this area is oily, a common condition even if the rest of your face is dry.

- **Look at your hairline.** Do you see any blemishes, blackheads, tiny bumps, or skin eruptions? These can be caused by excessive use of hair spray, gels, or pomades, or by perspiration or the styling of hair onto your forehead.

- **Focus for a minute on your chin.** Look for bumps under the skin or tiny blackheads. Oily skin can be aggravated by bacteria coming from a telephone receiver or the palm of your hand, two unexpected but frequent causes of breakouts in the chin area.

- **Do you wear glasses?** If you do on an everyday basis, take a closer look at the sides and bridge of your nose, where your glasses touch your skin. If you see tiny eruptions here, you may not be cleaning your glasses often enough—which should be, like your skin, a minimum of twice a day, morning and night.

- **Watch for these signs of skin that is sensitive.** Whether your skin is dry, oily, or combination, look out for red blotches, broken capillaries, fine spidery lines, and isolated flakiness.

Don't be concerned if you don't like what you have just seen! I have yet to meet a single person, during all my years in the skin care business, who was 100 percent happy with the way his or her skin looked. Even those of us who are not at all concerned with our appearance will note the passage of time in our faces, will suddenly see the results of one too many contacts with the extremes of Mother Nature. Bear in mind too: No one else looks at your skin through a magnifying glass, and for the most part, everything you are seeing now can be improved with the help of the information contained within this book.

OUR SKIN HISTORY: NATURE PLUS NURTURE

Be aware that your skin is, in many ways, a road map not merely of your contact with the environment but of your genetic past. Granted, many of us reflect the influences of a "melting pot" heritage, but there are many remaining influences of our primary genetic pasts. In general, skin can be divided into four major cultural groups: White, Black, Hispanic, and Oriental. Bear in mind that these are very general observations based on my contact with many different clients over the years. Some factors within your category may not apply to you, while you may also have influences from several categories.

White skin   This falls into two basic subgroups: **fair** (Nordic/British) and **olive** (Mediterranean). Fair skin is light in color, thin in texture, and highly vulnerable to dryness, broken capillaries, and environmental damage from wind and sun. Olive skin tends to be oilier, more prone to blackheads and, by virtue of its darker pigment, has more natural protection against sun- and windburn.

Black skin   While its cells contain a higher concentration of pigment (melanin) than white skin, black skin is **not**—as many blacks erroneously perceive—immune to the hazards of sun-induced aging and skin cancer. Black skin needs protection, although what it may not need is the addition of heavy creams and oils.

A common misconception is that all black skin is oily. While the vast majority of blacks do have skin with a natural tendency to be oily, 5 percent of my black clients actually have extremely dry complexions, which often show up in ashy, gray-looking patches. Many black men with normal or

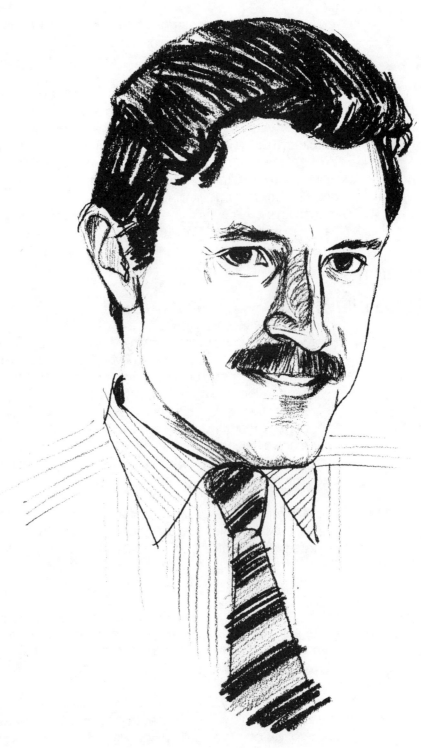

In grooming, it's the details that count.

combination skin create overoily skin by slathering on heavy oil-based lotions each morning.

A common and often painful problem afflicting many black men is ingrown hairs, caused by the tendency of a curly hair to grow back down into the hair follicle rather than straight out of the skin surface. This problem can be exacerbated by shaving and by the mistaken use of home treatments that cause further skin infection rather than serving as a cure. (Because this is such a widespread problem, I have devoted an entire section of the shaving chapter to dealing with ingrown hairs.)

Hispanic skin   This type of skin is rarely dry, usually combination or oily. Hispanic men who have sensitive skin may find that a diet that reflects their cultural heritage (one that is rich in spicy or fried foods) can aggravate preexisting skin problems. While Hispanics tend to have olive-toned complexions that tan rather than burn when exposed to sunlight, their skin still needs to be protected from the sun's damaging rays.

Oriental skin   This type of skin tends to have a smooth surface that, much like Oriental hair, beautifully reflects the light. What is also common among Orientals, though, is highly sensitive skin. Once it becomes acne- or blemish-prone, it tends to heal very slowly over periods of weeks rather than days. Oriental men may also find during shaving that their skin will succumb to nicks or cuts that also heal more slowly than similar abrasions in their white-skinned counterparts.

Note: The darker your skin, the more you need to be aware of the possibilities of hyperpigmented (or dark-toned) scarring, and the more careful you must be to avoid self-treatment of acne blemishes. Just as your skin's melanocytes (or pigmenting cells) are better able to rush to the skin surface to protect your skin from sun damage, so too can they rush to protect your skin from other perceived "attacks," such as the assault of squeezing or picking at a blemish. The major consequence: unlike a suntan, a pigmented scar will not fade away and, in fact, can grow more obvious over time. (More on skin scarring and how to avoid it in Chapter 4.)

BEYOND THE SURFACE:
YOUR SKIN'S INNER WORKINGS

Obviously, what we have just been discussing is the skin you can see, the skin that is visible to all as you walk down the street, eat in a restaurant, talk at a business meeting. But what determines the appearance of the skin's surface begins underneath, in the layers of the skin that cannot be seen with the naked eye.

THE SKIN: THE BODY'S LARGEST ORGAN

The skin of an adult covers approximately 18 square feet and weighs an average of 6 pounds or more. It varies in thickness from the thinnest, most delicate skin of the eyelids to the thicker, more rugged skin of the soles of the feet and palms of the hands.

Every inch of skin contains millions of cells, along with sensory nerve endings and networks of vital blood vessels. The skin also contains about three million tiny sweat glands that go to work when the body begins to register an increase in inner or outer heat. Each square inch of skin also contains a multitude of tiny hairs, many so fine they can be seen only with a magnifying glass, others—as in the beard and scalp areas—more than easily obvious to the unaided eye.

Three Main Layers

The skin is divided into three main layers. The outermost layer, the one that is visible to us, is the **epidermis**. The topmost portion of this layer is composed of dead, rather than living, skin cells that are continually in the process of flaking away and being renewed by new cells from underneath. When we are young and vigorous, this is a smooth process; as we age, like all body functions, this shedding can become slower and sluggish, and need outside assistance to be "speeded up." Also within the epidermis are found the openings of the hair follicles and sweat glands commonly known as pores. The deepest layer of the epidermis is known as the germinative or basal cell layer; it is within this layer that new epidermal cells are formed and begin their journey to the outermost skin surface. These cells are also the repository of the skin's pigment (or melanin), our body's natural protection factor against some, but not all, of the hazards of the sun.

The second-deepest skin layer is the **dermis**. The dermis is primarily composed of the fibrous protein known as collagen, the same substance that gives skin its integrity, its shape, and its flexibility. When damaged by the sun's rays and the passage of time the dermis begins to break down and "stretch out," and eventually it forms the undesirable sags that show up on the surface as wrinkles. Within the dermis are also whole networks of blood vessels, nerves, oil and sweat glands, as well as the "roots" of hair follicles. The nerve endings within the dermis are highly sophisticated, able to detect subtle differences in heat and cold, pain or pressure, as well as vibration and movement.

The skin's innermost layer is known as the **subcutaneous tissue.** Composed primarily of fatty, or adipose, cells, this layer is the body's ultimate insulator and also gives the skin its smooth shape and contour. The amount of fat found in this layer, and its actual thickness, varies not only from one man to the next but also changes from one part of the body to another—a result of body type as well as genetics and heredity. Age, sex, and general health all affect the fatty layer's thickness, but one thing is certain: If this fatty

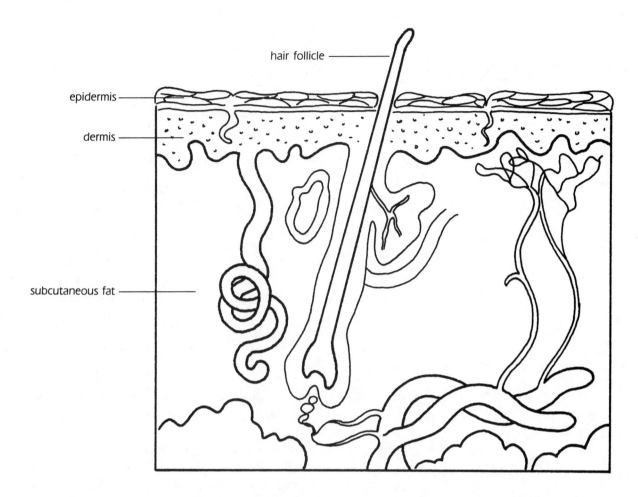

hair follicle —

epidermis —

dermis —

subcutaneous fat —

cushion becomes too thin, the body loses its ability to regulate its own temperature, to function at a normal level, and to carry on regular body processes. While it may be true that a man can never be too rich, it is not true, from the standpoint of health and vitality, that he can never be too thin!

WEATHERING THE SEASONS

You have just read how the inner workings of the skin contribute to its outer appearance. It is important, along with inner skin science, to remember that we live in an ever-changing, never-static environment, and that skin is the body's primary contact with the world around us. The majority of Americans enjoy the changing climates of four uniquely different seasons; all too often they expose their skin to unrecognized hazards of temperature and humidity extremes. Whether you are an avid outdoorsman or an equally avid stay-at-home, chances are your skin must adapt to several shifts of indoor and outdoor environments throughout every year of your life. Let's look at the changing seasonal demands the weather makes on your skin, and some general advice on weathering all of the various seasons.

17

SUMMER SUNTIME

For most men, summer means more time spent outdoors, more perspiration, and less skin hydration. Adding to this problem are: the dry air indoors, the result of the cooling pleasures of air conditioning, and closed-tight office windows. Whatever your skin type, you need to increase your daily intake of cool, clear water to help hydrate your skin from the inside out, as well as to increase your use of water-based lotions and moisturizers to help hold this extra moisture inside your skin cells, to help your skin stay "plumped-up" and healthy looking.

Summer sun means pleasurable days playing tennis, relaxing on beaches and backyard lawns. It also can mean increased exposure to the sun's ultraviolet rays, now proven beyond a doubt to be the number-one cause of premature aging of the skin, as well as a causative factor in the development of skin cancer. Protection is the key and, thanks to new advances in sunscreening agents, it is also easier—and more comfortable— than ever. (See Chapter 6 for a full rundown on the sun and your skin, and Chapter 11 for skin-saving ways of "faking" a tan year-round.)

For Dry Skin: Watch for skin parching and flaking; adding a cup of warm milk to a warm bath can help smooth skin dryness.

For Oily Skin: Breakouts can be exacerbated by perspiration during hot weather, so be sure to cleanse skin thoroughly, especially after outdoor exercise.

If your skin feels sluggish and your muscles feel a little sore from warm-weather overexertion, consider the skin-stimulating pleasures of the following summer-refresher.

Mid-summer Zinger:
Ginger Bath

Grate a large ginger root and steep it in boiling water for 20 minutes. Strain the mixture. Add the liquid to a tubful of warm (**not** hot) water. Place the grated ginger in a washcloth and tie it closed with a rubber band. Use this "spice sponge" to cleanse skin gently (don't rub the skin; it's not a linoleum floor) and "rev up" circulation.

On particularly hot humid days, use talcum powder (perhaps fragranced in your favorite after shave scent, as now widely available) to reduce friction between your skin and clothes. Try to allow yourself extra time to get from one place to the next, so you're not rushing around in the heat. Remember to allow time for all-important relaxation. If you do perspire, as is inevitable, remember that the sooner you can cleanse it off your skin, the better. For example, if your job requires many trips in and out of the office during the day, consider keeping a washcloth and gentle cleanser in your desk drawer for midday facial cleansing. Not only will it help improve the look of your skin, it will also lift your spirits, help you feel cleaner, fresher all over—certainly a desirable goal in the heat of a hot summer day!

FALL: THE MOISTURE FACTOR

As the air gets cooler, it also gets drier. The colder the air, the less its ability to hold moisture—and the greater its tendency to "rob" water from available sources, like your skin. At this time of year, your face and body start requiring additional "moisture attention," especially if you've gotten a bit too much sun during the summer and are experiencing post-summer skin flaking or peeling.

For Dry Skin: To increase your skin's moisture level, hook up a humidifier in your office **and** at home. Pace your day with water breaks, drinking six-to-eight glasses daily. Get into the "double-dose routine" of applying moisturizer right after shaving, waiting ten minutes, and reapplying; this is a moisture-saver that you should practice right through the winter.

If soap is leaving your skin flaky and dull after cleansing, consider a switch to a cream- or gel-formula cleanser instead, to remove surface dirt without stripping skin of its natural, essential oils. Always use lukewarm, not hot, water for cleansing.

For Oily Skin: Rather than using harsh alcohol-based astringents (often called toners), consider a nonalcohol-based version, either a commercially-available formula or a recipe I keep in my refrigerator all year long to remove excess oil and to give your skin a fresh-cooled feeling.

Lettuce Essence Lotion

Find the darkest-leaved lettuce you can. Boil leaves in enough water to cover. Let cool and strain. Add the juice of one cucumber. Refrigerate. Apply all over face after cleansing; use sterile cotton rather than more irritating tissue to apply.

For Combination Skin: Don't overlook skin's dry patches, whether high on the cheekbones or under the eyes. A moisturizer formulated with allantoin or cocoa butter is a good choice.

For All Skin Types: The start of colder weather is also the beginning of the chapped-lip and dry-hands season. Carry a stick-formula lip balm in your briefcase or suit jacket pocket and use it daily. If your lips crack, don't pull or pick at them; allow the skin to heal naturally while keeping it moisturized. Hands require daily moisturizing, morning and night, as well as following each hand-washing if at all possible. Avoid using harsh commercial soaps, which tend to overdry the skin.

WINTER COLD WATCH

Cold, dry air and harsh, stinging winds make winter one of the roughest seasons for your skin to endure. If you're heading outdoors for any length of time, the kindest step you can take for your skin is to wear a knitted wool face mask, with cutouts for your eyes, nostrils, and mouth—and leave vanity behind!

For Dry and Combination Skin: Be especially wary of the windchill factor. A windburn can be as painful as—and sometimes take longer to heal than—a sunburn. Try not to shave right before going outdoors when it's especially cold or windy, as this can further irritate the skin. Double up on the amount of moisturizer and lip balm you apply, waiting five minutes between applications. **Never** use alchol-based shave products at this time of year.

For Oily Skin: Even men with oily complexions usually notice some dry, flaky patches around the edge of the nostrils, near the eyebrows, on the edges of he cheeks by midwinter. It is important that you use a moisturizer on these areas on a daily basis, but stick to a water-based lotion or light cream formula to avoid clogging the pores and causing blemishes. Even men who use soap to wash their faces in summer will probably want to switch to a cream-formula cleanser at this time of year to avoid overdrying the skin.

For All Skin Types: Remember that dry skin doesn't necessarily stop at the face. After shaving, don't forget to moisturize your neck along with your facial skin. To avoid chapping of arms, legs, and body skin, shower or bathe no more than once a day (unless, of course, you've been working up a heavy sweat at the gym) and always apply body cream afterward. The bath water should be no warmer than 104°F. Avoid overly-long soaking in winter; it can strip your skin of protective oils. Use a moisture-restoring body cleanser (many of the new liquid shower/bath-body shampoos contain extra moisturizing ingredients) instead of harsh detergent soaps. If your skin becomes excessively red and scaly (say on elbows, knees), apply a small amount of baby oil after the bath or shower while skin is still damp.

Beware of scalp dryness during winter, which is often mistaken for dandruff but is actually dry skin. Wear a hat outdoors to protect the scalp from cold, dry air. Apply conditioner after every shampo, rubbing it into the scalp gently right before the final rinsing **only** if your scalp is excessively dry. In winter, you needn't wash your hair every day unless your hair is very oily or you have been exercising and working up a sweat.

If you like the relaxation of a sauna, switch to a steam room instead. It is less drying for the skin, especially important in winter. When you do use a sauna, whatever the time of year, try not to stay in more than five minutes at a time, and don't let the temperature exceed 110°F.

SPRING GROOMING

Spring. For people as well as plants, this is a season of reawakening and renewal. The cold of winter has given way to more warmth, more sunshine, more energy. People everywhere feel more alive, more awake, than ever. If you treat yourself to a salon facial only once a year, this is the time of year to choose, when a skin care expert can cleanse away the accumulated dry skin of winter, and help prepare your skin for the outdoor pleasures—and skin dangers—of summer to come.

In any case, this is the season that is kindest to your skin. There are no extremes of temperature outdoors, nor air conditioning or heat indoors. The weather is perfect for walking, jogging, bicycling, and other activities, and your skin has the perfect chance to "rebalance" itself without any outside stresses.

For Dry Skin: This is the time of year your skin will naturally look its best. You may notice that you need a less greasy moisturizer and can cut down on the number of times you apply it daily. In other words, you can spend less time on your skin and more time enjoying springtime's pleasures.

For Combination and Oily Skin: Spring's gentle climate often provides relief from extremes of oiliness and dryness, and helps even out the look and texture of your skin. This doesn't mean you should forget about your skin care routine; it just means you'll often find the climate more conducive to keeping oily patches at bay. If you do need to apply a light moisturizer lotion, avoid the T-zone area (nose and forehead).

Whatever your skin type, if you can't make it to a skin care specialist, but want to do something special to welcome the season and soothe and smooth your skin, consider the skin refreshment of my special **Mélange Mask.**

Mélange Mask

Mix together 3 teaspoons of beer, 1 teaspoon of plain unflavored yogurt, ½ teaspoon of lemon juice, 2 teaspoons of orange juice, 2 teaspoons of grated carrot, and a few drops of olive oil (use sparingly if your skin is oily). Apply to the face and leave on for ten minutes. (You might want to take this time to put your feet up and close your eyes and relax.) Rinse thoroughly with lukewarm water; pat skin dry with a clean towel.

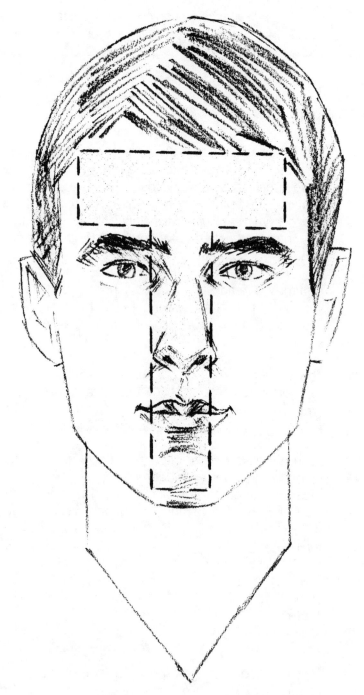

Where skin is oiliest: the "T-zone."

CHAPTER THREE

SKIN CARE AT EVERY AGE

He that is not handsome at 20, nor strong at 30, nor rich at 40, nor wise at 50, will never be handsome, strong, rich or wise.

—George Herbert (1593-1633)

At every stage of your life, there are three reasons for you to visit a skin care expert: to learn about your skin, to relax, and to help you continue to look the best you can. The skin is, in many ways, a mirror of a man's vitality and health. You can wear the most impeccably-tailored clothing, have the perfect haircut, the ultimate in fine leather shoes, belts, and accessories, but if you're not happy with the look of your skin, chances are you won't be pleased with your overall appearance. Here's the best news of all: It is never too early or too late to begin taking care of your skin. Once you make skin care a regular habit, it will not only improve your looks, but it will help to increase your self-confidence for the rest of your life. Science has increasingly proven it: When we feel that we look good, we feel better about ourselves—and other people react more positively to us as well.

More and more American men are realizing what their European counterparts have known for years: Good grooming involves more than ducking into the corner barbershop for a "shave 'n a haircut." In my native country of Israel, the harsh year-round sunlight forces everyone, male and female, to be more aware of skin care, lest we all end up brown and wrinkled as raisins well before middle-age. Yet even in the more temperate climate of America, the skin is exposed to extremes of environment that take their toll as the years pass by. Add in the emotional ups and downs, as well as the biological and hormonal changes that occur in every man's life as he grows from puberty to adulthood, and you begin to see that the skin has a good deal to contend with. Like other good habits, skin care is a routine that is most easily established when a man is relatively young.

MAKING IT THROUGH PUBERTY

If you are lucky enough to have passed through the early teen years with clear skin, then thank your guardian angel for the good fortune. As a noted dermatologist once said in a lecture on teenage acne, "As if it isn't difficult enough to make it through the emotional maze of early adolescence, to cope with pants that are suddenly two inches too short and find an identity you can call your own, our bodies have to throw in the double whammy of playing havoc with the oiliness and blemish production of our skin."

For the young male teenager who is dealing with the increased growth and hormonal production of his body and trying to come to terms with this new being known as his "self," even an occasional blemish or pimple seems like a huge, overgrown blot on his skin that must be visible for miles. The last person he feels comfortable discussing the state of his skin with is usually Dad.

About 15 percent of my salon clientele are teenagers. Most of them, girls as well as boys, are first brought there somewhat unwillingly by their mothers. Even though Mom means well, the first thing I do is to ask her to step aside, to wait outside during the initial consultation, so the teenager and I can talk freely. The young man tells me a little about himself, about the kind of life he leads, whether he has any hobbies or favorite sports, and about how much time he is willing to devote to his skin. If we hit it off during this initial consultation, then I know this is a boy I can help. If he spends the whole time he's supposed to be talking to me being angry with his mother for dragging him in to see me to begin with, then I tell him there is little that I can do for him—although this latter scenario, I have found, is rarely the case. Usually once the two of us begin talking, the young man finds I am a great deal less threatening, and a good deal more sensible, than he thought.

One point I must make here: While a skin care expert can help a young man who has oily skin and an occasional acne blemish to keep his breakouts under control, no skin care expert should treat severe cystic acne that covers the entire face, which requires the types of prescription medications only a dermatologist can provide. Beware of overzealous skin care salons claiming that there is no problem they cannot cure. While there is often a fine line between problems treated by qualified skin care specialists and dermatologists, in general, acne that is made up of numerous inflamed cysts will require at least preliminary treatment by a doctor, who may then approve of follow-up skin cleansing by a skin care expert. General skin oiliness accompanied by occasional, noninflamed or infected blemishes can be successfully treated by a well-trained skin care specialist. (For a full discussion of oily skin and acne, see the following chapter.) As in most skin care questions, the key to finding the proper treatment is a good dose of common sense—both yours and the skin care salon staff's! If you feel too much is being promised, then go elsewhere.

THE TEEN YEARS

This is the time of life when every young man wants to be independent, and every parent, no matter how open-minded, has a tendency to try to hold on to "my little boy." While 90 percent of my 16-year-old clients originally visit my salon due to their parents' concerns about skin rather than their own, the majority of men who begin visiting my salon for basic skin care advice in their teen years become my clients (and friends) for life. The reason: I make it clear to them that I am here to help them, to ease their worries about their skin, to make skin care less—not more—complicated, and to share my knowledge with them, **not** to lecture them on skin care.

My teenage clients accept me as an authority figure because I offer them moral support as well as advice. I understand their concern for their appearance is only a part of their total personalities, but that it is an especially fragile part during the difficult teenage years, when all of us—men and women—are intent on looking our best while pretending we don't give a darn!

The teen years are the perfect years to develop a common-sense attitude to skin care. Here are some important facts to learn now, and remember throughout your life:

- **Don't pick at your face.** Tiny scars you cause now will last forever. As you age and your skin stretches or sags, what are virtually invisible scars now can become much more obvious as they stretch and enlarge with the surrounding skin. In the long run, getting rid of these scars may involve a skin "planing" technique like dermabrasion or chemical peel, or a "puffing-up" treatment like collagen injections (these are described in Chapter 11).

- **Keep your nails and hands clean.** Not only do clean hands and nails look more refined and more attractive, they also help to prevent the spread of bacteria to your delicate facial skin. While we all know we shouldn't touch our hands to our face, sometimes it's easy to unconsciously cradle our chins in our hands; the cleaner our hands are, the clearer our skin will stay.

- **Treat a skin problem professionally when it's small.** Rather than experimenting with cleansers, lotions, and potions yourself, discuss small problems with an expert whenever possible to avoid transforming a small problem into a major one by misguided at-home skin care. You may not require a salon treatment, but remember that consultations are an important part of the services rendered by skin care specialists. One way to judge an expert is not only by the efficacy of his or her treatments but by the validity of his or her advice, and the degree of concern he or she shows for helping you to take care of your skin at home. If there aren't any skin care salons nearby, don't overlook complimentary consultations available at department store men's skin care counters. Look for someone who is more than a salesperson, though, and has had some skin science training. Better yet, consult a pharmacist who can provide advice on nonprescription skin preparations.

• **Be aware that skin care does not have to be time-consuming.** The biggest complaint from teenage boys: "I don't want to spend hours in front of the mirror like my sister or my mom." There's no reason to. If your skin is basically healthy, all I'll advise is to switch from using harsh soap on your face to using a cleansing lotion, and to apply a moisturizer to your skin where it's dry. In fact, these days I am surprised by how many of my male clients ask me for more products than I advise that they need!

• **Be aware of the diet/skin health connection.** While there are no magic foods that will guarantee freedom from blemishes, and no foods ever proven beyond a doubt to cause breakouts, there is growing scientific evidence that a healthful diet contributes to a sound, healthy body. Take time out to eat real meals, not just snacks. Trade the quick energy/quick let-down of junk foods for the high-energy, high-vitality of a well-balanced diet (see Chapter 7).

THE STRESS-FILLED TWENTIES

These are the years of rapid changes, from going off to college to live away from your family for the first time, to college graduation and going out into the world as an adult. Your image, your personal presentation suddenly become important as you go out on job interviews, do your first sales call, meet your business associates and customers for the first time. Your skin may not have changed much since your teens, but chances are you look in the mirror a little more often and a little more carefully these days, as you get ready to face a new world of challenge and opportunity each morning.

Daily shaving is a habit most men begin at the same time they begin their first job. Learning to shave properly involves more than deciding how much to spend on a razor; it involves learning to protect your skin from the daily onslaught, to use the products that will help your razor glide over, rather than slice at, your skin. For this reason, I've devoted an entire chapter to the subjet of shaving—and suggest every man develop a good shaving routine as early in life as he can (see Chapter 5).

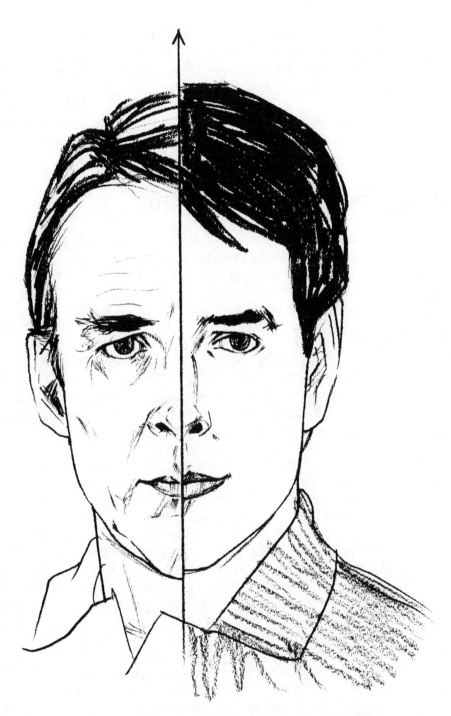

Aging's first targets: the skin around the eyes and mouth.

Be aware at this age that this is the perfect time to begin building toward the future, not just in terms of setting up solid financial records, establishing a good credit rating, learning about business and developing a career path, but in more personal matters, too. This is a time of exploration, meeting new friends, dating, buying new clothes appropriate to your job, and beginning to make an investment in the health and appearance of your skin. One of the best things you can buy yourself now is a good sunscreen, the best protection your skin can **ever** have.

THE ACHIEVEMENT-ORIENTED THIRTIES

These are the "go-go" years, when your job, your relationships, and your family are on the move. By this time, many men have married, bought a co-op apartment or a house, and have a family that they are watching and helping to grow. These are also years when you feel a bit more established, have time to develop more confidence in yourself and your abilities, and to set goals for yourself and for your loved ones.

In terms of your skin, this is the time when the most subtle signs of aging may just be beginning to appear—and when the commitment to skin care is most important of all.

At this age, I see some panic-stricken men in my salon. "Help!" they say. "I woke up this morning, looked in the mirror, and saw tiny lines around my eyes." Or, "I just realized that the tiny lines around my mouth I see when I smile don't all go away when I stop smiling." While I can't promise these men eternal youth—and while they frequently exaggerate the degree of wrinkling that has actually taken place in their skin—I can help these men to develop habits that will keep their skin looking their best right now and during the many active years to come.

The first skin care rule of the thirties: You must begin using some type of eye cream now. Even if you think your skin doesn't show any signs of aging, the delicate skin of the eye area, which contains little or no oil glands, is beginning to lose its elasticity now. It needs help from outside in staving off moisture loss and keeping the "plumpness" we associate with youthful skin. What's more, the eyes are the first feature we notice, the face's most vivid spot of communication. When we have a conversation, we look each other in the eyes. You should begin using a light, moisture-rich eye cream, one that is refreshingly cool-feeling on the skin and that can be nourishing to your skin and help soothe and "brighten" tired eyes each day. Apply eye cream morning and night, after you wash your face and splash on a cool-water rinse.

THE "MIDLIFE CRUNCH" FORTIES

From many a woman's point of view, a man in his forties is eminently attractive. Established in his career, aware of his inner strength and intelligence, he should be feeling on top of the world, right? Perhaps for some men, but for others, the forties are the years of "midlife crisis," when a man feels his first tinge of mortality, has doubts about his security, fears of inferiority, loss of masculinity and increased vulnerability.

Men in their forties see one wrinkle and fear five will follow. They see small lines that are inevitable at this age (unless you've lived in a vacuum-sealed package all your life) and fear their looks are deserting them.

Now **is** the time to take an honest—and by this I mean logical, not paranoid—look at your skin. You really can't fool Mother Nature anymore. This is the time of life when, in general, your body stops bouncing back from punishment as quickly as before. No longer can you drink too much alcohol, sleep too little, smoke too many cigarettes or take too many drugs without it showing up in a certain gray cast to your skin or a look of bloodshot redness in your eyes. If your body weight tends to fluctuate, no longer will your skin easily stretch and retighten as the scale moves up and down. In fact, every skin care expert will advise you: If you need to lose weight, do so when you're young and keep it off. Not only is it healthier in general; it's also the only way to avoid seeing a certain laxity in your skin as it fails to fully "redrape" itself on your newly-slimmed frame. At 40, your skin begins losing some of its elasticity, no matter how well you've cared for it up to now.

This is not to suggest that working to stay in shape isn't worth it at this age. It is most certainly worthwhile caring for your skin, keeping your weight down, exercising and working out more. It's just that, more than ever, what you need to look your best now and in the future comes from inside as well as outside: a young spirit, a sense of vitality, a healthy dose of realism tempered with a zest for life.

In clients of this age I see a real appreciation, perhaps for the first time ever, of what skin care can mean for the psyche as well as for the appearance. They tell me, "Coming in for a facial is one of the few times I get to relax, to do something totally for myself, to feel the pressure is off." When they leave the salon, not only does their skin look cleaner, but it literally looks more relaxed. When a man feels the tension leave his mind and body, he carries himself with more ease, walks with a freer jaunt, looks more attractive. Needing to relax is nothing to feel guilty about; in fact, scientists are learning it is essential to being a healthy human being, and can help you live a longer, more complete life (see the chapter on stress later in this book).

THE FABULOUS FIFTIES

If a man has taken care of his skin and stayed out of the sun, there is no reason his skin should look any older at 50 than it did at 40. Yet, who among us can totally resist the lure, and allure, of a suntan, of long afternoons of sailing and sunning, of skiing vacations or trips to the shore? At 50, a man's skin reflects the best—and the worst—of his life!

A man has going for him the fact that his naturally thicker skin and lack of abrupt hormonal shift into menopause will keep him looking younger longer than a woman of the same age. In fact, many plastic surgeons report that their male patients are an average of ten years older than their female patients (see the section on plastic surgery in Chapter 11).

Some factors that will also help you make a smoother transition into your sixties: The inner support of living a full and satisfying life, learning to take the good times with the bad, and a wife and family who love you and are loved by you. You'll also be better off if you've learned to take time out to relax—one of the key benefits of the pampering of a skin care salon.

It is rare for oily skin to persist into the fifties. It is more common for skin to become somewhat drier, and more flaky, and for sensitive skin to become even more so. A skin care expert can help you adjust your skin care routine to the new needs of your skin, and to be aware of changes that may signify the treatment you are using is not quite right.

At this age, sun protection is more essential than ever. It won't undo the aging process (nothing can), but it can prevent the more concentrated, intense skin damage that can occur at this age, when your skin is not able to repair or regenerate itself as quickly as when you were younger—and when the collagen fibers within the skin are already beginning to lose a good deal of their natural firmness and strength.

Most men come to a skin care salon now to see if they can look younger but also simply to relax—to "escape" on a mini-vacation where the phones aren't ringing, the demands of business are on hold, where the focus is oneself and the stress is off. Clients who visit my salon for the first time in their fifties often exclaim: "If I'd ever known how relaxing a facial could be, I'd have been coming here for years." A man in his fifties knows I'm not giving him his youth back; he is happy, though, that I'm giving him his sense of balance and relaxation back simply by focusing pampering attention on him.

Many men in their fifties do a good deal of traveling for business and pleasure. Here are some simple tips to offset the drying effect frequent plane travel can have on the skin.

• **Before boarding the plane,** apply a slightly creamy moisturizer, even if your skin is oily. The air inside a plane is kept very dry to maintain cleanliness; this also means that moisture will be drawn out of the upper layers of your skin and into the air throughout the plane trip. If you arrive for your flight early or are kept waiting in the lounge area due to a travel delay, drink a tall glass of water or club soda to boost your interior moisture reserves. Avoid alcohol- or caffeine-containing drinks as these actually decrease body liquid stores in the long run.

• **During plane travel,** utilize the time to read, watch a movie, and listen to music tapes, but don't stay glued to your seat for hours on end. Get up and walk around a bit, do some unobtrusive stretching exercises in your seat, anything to keep your muscles from becoming lax and more fatigued. To keep your skin and spirits refreshed, rinse your face with cool water every few hours or so, then reapply a light layer of moisturizer. On a long trip, ask the steward or stewardess to bring you some cold cotton compresses about an hour or two before landing (or tuck cotton balls into your carry-on bag and make your own). Close your eyes for ten minutes, apply the compresses, and you'll wake up feeling more refreshed.

Also important: drink plenty of water, avoid alcohol and caffeine whenever possible, and eat lightly (salad, fruit, and bread rather than meat and gloppy potatoes) in order to feel at your best when the plane lands.

• **On arrival,** try not to rush around immediately if you can avoid it. Adjust your skin care to the new environment, using "lighter" products if it's hot and humid, "heavier" richer moisturizers if it's cold and dry. Whenever possible, discuss your travel schedule with your skin care expert before you go. That way, you can bring along smaller, travel-size versions of the products you'll need, to make packing/unpacking easier, allow you to travel light, and have minimal shopping needs in a strange city.

THE SUPER SIXTIES

If you've been skin-smart—and lucky enough to have parents who passed along genes for youthful-looking skin—you'll find that at 60 you barely look 50! For most men, the sixties are a time for enjoying life more, for beginning to rate relaxation as more of a life priority, and for recognizing that, even if you can't do and have it all, there's certainly a lot around you that brings you pleasure. Today a man of 60 is more likely to be found in the gym working out after a day at the office than he is to be lounging in front of the television set—and his appearance has the vitality that reflects this shift.

At this age, you'll find that a skin care expert can't make drastic changes in your appearance. What we can do, and what is equally, if not more, important, is to help you to keep looking your best, to feel good about yourself, and to relax. We can help you make the right choices in skin care and help you avoid spurious claims of "magic" anti-wrinkle cures. For many of my clients who have been coming to skin care salons for years, reaching their sixties marks a change in their attitude toward skin care. They consider the relaxation and the time alone to be as vital to the look **and** feel of their skin as the actual cleansing and replenishing treatments. In many ways, they're right.

THE SEVENTIES AND BEYOND

Believe it or not, one of my most loyal clients is a man who recently celebrated his 74th birthday. I would never dare claim that at this point in his life I am doing very much to alter his appearance, but he tells me that what counts is that I make him **feel** ageless once a month, even if he can't look it! Judging by his spirit and energy, I expect to keep seeing this man in my salon every month for years to come—and who am I to argue with such a testimonial?

Men today are living longer, staying active longer, and enjoying life longer than ever before. We all—men and women—know more about preventive medicine and about taking care of our bodies than past generations even dreamed possible. And we are all looking, and feeling, the better for it.

FACIAL EXERCISES?

We all know by now that exercise does wonders for body shape, decreases body fat, and gives skin more sleekness and tone (see Chapter 9). But can individual facial exercises make a difference in the tone and shape of our faces? The evidence, alas, is not all in. There are some experts who claim miraculous results from facial exercise routines, while there are others who claim that they are a total waste of time and that, in some cases, these exercises may create more new wrinkles than they "erase." What does seem apparent, though, is that facial exercises cannot cure wrinkles or sags. Once you look old, plastic surgery is going to do a great deal more for you than facial exercises—although good skin care can help you learn how to camouflage a great deal of premature wrinkling, even if it can't do away with lines and sagging skin.

The bottom line is that facial exercises may not cure wrinkles, but they probably can't hurt, either—and they **can** make your face **feel** more alive and refreshed. Here are the exercises I provide for clients in my salon who want to give them a try.

Start out slowly. If an exercise seems difficult, repeat it fewer times than I've suggested, then work up to the total number of repetitions. Remember, you may be using muscles you rarely use, so what seems like it should be easy to do may feel difficult the first few times.

Chin-and-Neck Firmer: Lie down on a bed with your head hanging over the edge. Clench your jaw until the cords of the neck stand out. Open and close mouth five times.

Keeping jaws clenched and teeth closed, **slowly** raise your head to an upright position, then drop slowly. Repeat five times.

Letting your head hang, gently twist it first to the right, then to the left. Do ten times.

Kiss-and-Smile: Stand in an upright position. Drop head back, pucker lips, and stretch nose toward the ceiling. Slowly release your lips and grin as wide as you can. Repeat five times.

Lower Lip-and-Chin Firmer: Stand in an upright position. Drop head back, push lower lip out in a pout as far as you can, feeling for the stretch in your neck muscles. Release the lower lip, still keeping neck and jaw taut. Slowly raise your head and release muscles. Repeat five times.

Upper Cheek Strengthener: Flare your nostrils. Using clean fingers, push the pudgy part of the cheek upward. Tighten the cheek muscles under your fingers until the upper lip almost reaches your nose. Repeat five times.

Lower Cheek Strengthener: Holding lips together, smile slightly. Suck in the corners of your mouth, trying to bring your whole cheek in toward your teeth. Slowly release suction and smile. Repeat five times.

Upper-lip Firmer: Pucker lips in a kiss as tightly as possible. Slowly release and curl lips around your teeth (as in an exaggerated smile), while stretching the lips wide. When you've extended the lips as wide as possible, close your mouth and press your lips together. Repeat five times.

CHAPTER FOUR

ACNE: A SKIN TRIAL AT ANY AGE

The body is a test tube. You have to put in exactly the right ingredients to get the best reaction out of it.

—attributed to football player Jack Youngblood in **The Book of Quotes,** by Barbara Rowes (E.P. Dutton)

Everyone would like to have perfect skin, with bright, healthy-looking color and a smooth, clear surface. But the fact is that few of us, men or women, are lucky enough to have trouble-free complexions at any age, let alone throughout our lives. What also seems to be true is that skin troubles often crop up when we feel least able to cope with them, when our lives are filled with other stresses, or when we are undergoing some kind of emotional change or turmoil.

Between the ages of 12 and 20, when school, friends, and family pressures are often most intense, your chances of developing some type of skin blemish are well over 80 percent! And acne most commonly occurs in that 5 percent of the skin that we present to the world every day (the face) and at the age when our search for self-identification is most fragile.

Yet contrary to popular thought, acne is **not** merely a "teenage problem." It can persist not only into, but often doesn't even begin until, later in adulthood, when a man is in his twenties, thirties, or even forties. Despite the fact that acne treatment has undergone tremendous advances within the past decade—and that virtually **all** acne can be improved with proper therapy—there are still far too many men who needlessly endure the emotional pain and frustration of unattractive skin breakouts and unnecessary skin scarring.

MALE HORMONES: WHERE THE TROUBLE BEGINS

Although doctors still cannot predict who will get acne and who will not, they do agree that acne has some sort of hormonal connection, and that the culprits are male hormones (or androgens). Before puberty, oil glands are relatively inactive and blemishes are virtually nonexistent. With the onset of puberty, the body's hormonal production shifts, and the skin's sebaceous (or oil-producing) glands increase in both size and sebum (oil) output. While both men and women produce androgens, the amount of biologically-active male hormones are obviously much greater in men, a fact that probably accounts for the greater incidence of severe acne in men than in women.

Men with acne, however, do **not** have abnormally high levels of androgen hormones, nor are they oversexed or overaggressive or over-anything, note experts at The Dermatology Foundation. Men with acne do have more sebum secretion and higher amounts of acne-causing bacteria (know as Propionibacterium acnes or P. acnes). These bacteria have nothing at all to do with being dirty, but grow naturally within the ducts of the skin's oil glands as part of the interior chemistry of the skin. The reason for their overproduction and for the overproduction of sebum remain troubling mysteries for acne researchers, who are actively investigating such questions in laboratories around the world.

Also still puzzling acne experts: While severe acne seems to be hereditary in nature, it cuts across ethnic, cultural and generational lines. Eunuchs, who have underdeveloped sebaceous glands throughout life, do not develop acne, while women acne patients can be free of any type of hormonal imbalance. Seemingly conflicting this last fact but so far unexplainably: Even though they had no preexisting hormonal imbalance, women who take birth control pills often find as a side effect that their blemishes clear up.

THE GOOD NEWS: ACNE IS TREATABLE

The earlier treatment is begun the better, and the greater a man's chances of avoiding severe breakouts and unattractive skin scarring later in life. This is especially true in cases of teenage acne, often mistakenly viewed as a trivial concern, something to "grin and bear." If I can convince parents of a teenager of one thing, I hope it is that they should bring their son to a skin care expert at the first sign of an acne condition, to gain important information that will affect his appearance not only through his trying teen years but throughout the rest of his life. My reason here is not to promote my profession, but to avoid the most common skin disaster: that of an acne patient entering the office of a skin care expert or dermatologist with terrible, disfiguring skin scarring. Most of such scarring is the result not so much of the acne condition itself but of misguided attempts to clean it away at home. Overly rough cleansing and picking at the skin leads to the spread of skin infection, the

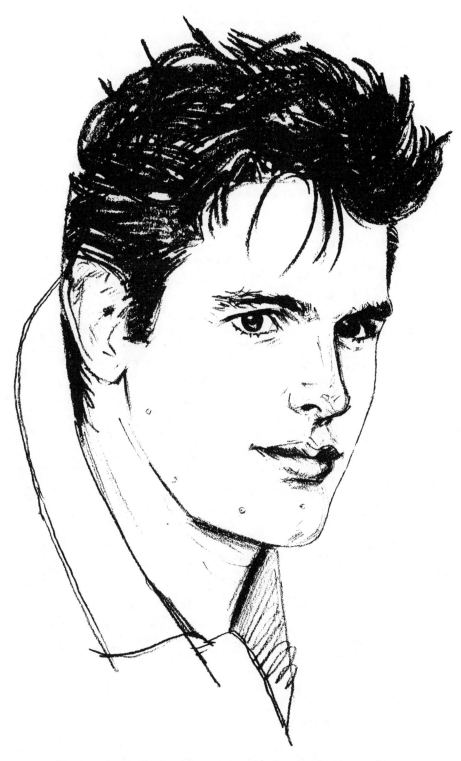

The best time to begin acne treatment is when breakouts are mild.

development of greater numbers of blemishes and, eventually, of pockmarked, pitted skin. How much easier and less traumatic to visit a skin care expert or dermatologist for a single consultation on proper skin cleansing technique, to educate the young man about his own responsibility for his skin's appearance and help him avoid all-too-common, all-too-indelible mistakes.

The goals of acne treatment are to lessen skin oiliness, clear up existing blemishes and, when possible, prevent future breakouts. These are aims that can be the province of a **well-trained** (and I emphasize this) skin care expert or of a dermatologist or, as in a growing number of major metropolitan areas, of a skin care team of the two professionals working together to promote clear, healthy skin.

The choice of who should treat your or your son's skin problem is an important and highly personal decision, but there are some basic guidelines I can offer. Whomever you go to for advice, be sure that acne is one of their special areas of expertise, and that they can speak logically and knowledgeably on the subject. Be aware that a skin care expert is likely to devote more time to very mild breakouts than is a physician, who is more concerned with true skin disease rather than more cosmetic problems. On the other hand, you need to know that severe cystic acne (characterized by inflamed, painful cysts under the skin that cover large skin areas, are red and bumpy) should always be brought to a physician's attention, as it is a problem that goes beyond a skin care expert's province to treat.

Whoever supervises your skin treatment, recognize that clearing up blemishes is not something done for you merely within the confines of a skin care salon or a dermatologist's office, but a process in which you have a vital role to play in terms of what you do and do not do at home. Be prepared to receive detailed at-home instructions and to follow them, or you will be wasting both your money and your time.

BREAKOUTS DEFINED

I am often asked by my clients to help them understand the different words used to describe acne blemishes, and will take a few moments here to define the terms most often used by dermatologists and other skin care experts. These words are not meant to intimidate, but to help you understand the physiological development of acne.

• **Blackheads** (or open comedones) are basically what we see of pore openings that have become clogged with a collection of dead skin cells, oil, and bacteria to such a degree that the walls of the pores become stretched and visible to the naked eye. The black-colored spot we see, rather than being caused by dirt as often supposed, is simply the deposition of skin

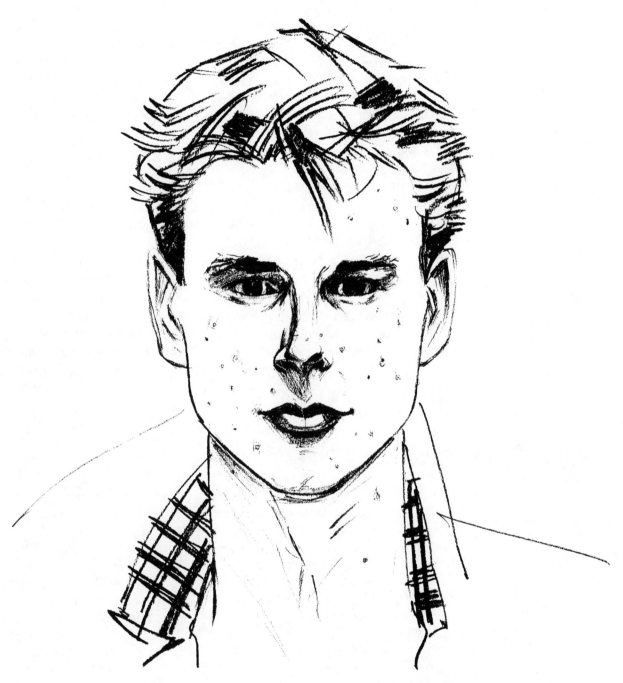

Modern medical advances mean there's hope even for severe acne.

pigment resulting from the interaction between the acne-causing bacteria and the dead skin cells.

• **Whiteheads** (or closed comedones) are small bumps that are either white or flesh-toned, and are basically blackheads that have developed further down under the surface of the skin. While blackheads often persist forever without changing, whiteheads are more often the precursors of more severe acne lesions.

• **Papules** are reddish bumps on the skin surface, often the next step after a whitehead. The red color indicates infection under the surface, and the body's effort to fight this infection by calling up white blood cells. It is at this stage that misguided picking and squeezing of papules can lead to spread of infection under the skin surface, and the emergence of additional unnecessary breakouts.

• **Pimples or pustules.** While the word pimple is often used by the layman to describe the full range of possible blemishes, dermatologists use this term to indicate a pus-filled, inflamed acne lesion.

• **Cystic acne** is the description of the widespread presence of highly-inflamed pimples, often in conjunction with the other types of blemishes described above. It is the most physically and emotionally severe type of acne. It is also the type of skin condition that should always be brought to a dermatologist's attention.

REAL HELP:
WHAT A GOOD SKIN CARE EXPERT CAN DO

My first words of advice are: Don't be discouraged, disgusted, or ashamed of your breakouts. They are a natural occurrence and can be greatly improved or even eliminated with proper skin treatments. In my years as a skin care expert, I have cleared up almost every acne problem I encountered, for roughly an 85 to 90 percent success rate. My only "failures" were in those men who, although they came to have regular salon treatments, cavalierly refused to follow my advice at home! Clearing up acne is a partnership, one in which I offer my expertise and understanding, in which I try to be a sensitive and caring listener as well as a guide, and in which I depend on your cooperation in following my advice at home. I am not saying that there is no case of acne that I cannot treat, but I will be more than honest in referring such cases to a qualified dermatologist.

• **What should you expect in the salon?** A skin exam and consultation should always be the first step. No diagnosis can be made without adequate information. A skin care expert needs to examine your skin, to view it closely under magnifying lenses and with the help of special lights, as well as to get your full medical history, learn about your diet, exercise, and skin care habits. The skin is an organ of the body, affected by the same factors as any other body part.

If you decide to have a facial, it should begin with gentle steaming and include a thorough-but-gentle pore cleansing, a drying mask (in my salon I use an Israeli Dead Sea-mud-based formula) and the application of drying lotion that soothes as well as absorbs oil from the skin.

• **How often do you need salon treatments?** This is a very individual question, but one that should be addressed during your initial visit, so that you can make an educated decision as to whether to commit yourself to the treatments. Many variables will affect the scheduling of your anti-acne treatments. For example, a man may have only a few surface blemishes but a good deal more acne activity under the skin surface. In that case, he may need to come to the salon as often as every other week for hour-long visits during the first two months, then cut back his visits to once every five-to-six weeks. A teenager whose acne is in a state of rapid spreading might benefit more by seeing a skin care expert for brief 20-minute visits once a week for several months, then come every other week for a while, and eventually come no more often than once a month. Whatever your particular case, one thing is clear: A good skin care expert or dermatologist should always give you some idea of the recommended treatment schedule during your initial consultation.

• **How long will it take to clear up your acne?** There is no one general answer here, but I do have some important advice: Beware of those specialists, whatever their reputation or credentials, who claim they can clear up your acne in less than three to four months. This does not mean that you won't see real improvement in the look of your skin before this time, or that inflammation and breakouts won't lessen greatly within even just a few weeks of a new skin care regime, but you cannot expect your skin condition, which was probably months or years in developing, to clear up overnight.

What you can and should expect is honesty. As I always tell my clients, "I can't perform miracles, but I can help you to help your skin to improve. If we both make a commitment to doing our best, I in the salon and you at home, chances are your skin will look a lot better, and you'll feel a lot better about yourself, within the next few months."

Equally important is that you don't need to wait forever to see your skin improve. After a few months of seeing a skin care expert or dermatologist, if your skin hasn't improved, ask the expert for an explanation. If you're not satisfied with the answer or the treatment you're receiving, go elsewhere. But be honest with yourself; no amount of high-quality professional care can undo mistreatment you may be giving your skin at home. Don't pick, rub, or scratch at your skin; the scarring you cause will counteract any possible benefits from seeking professional care.

AT-HOME CARE: KEY TO CLEAR SKIN

I've said it throughout this chapter: How you treat your skin at home on an everyday basis is the key to clearing up acne. Here are answers to the most common questions I get on this subject, and the advice I give to my private clients.

• **How should I clean my skin?** VERY GENTLY! I've told you that dirt does not cause acne, and scrubbing your skin will make the condition worse rather than better.

Even if you have only a single pimple, avoid using grainy cleansers, abrasive sponges, or even washcloths. These can all too easily break open a pimple and spread the infection to other areas of your face. Instead, use a gentle cleansing lotion specifically formulated for acne-prone skin (I recommend a sugar-based oil-absorbent fomula in my salon) applied with a clean cotton ball and rinsed with cool water (hot water cleansing tends to encourage further oil secretion).

• **Should I use an astringent? What kind?** An astringent is a light, clear or translucent liquid that restores skin's oil and moisture balance, removing any leftover cleansing lotion at the same time. Many men with acne-prone skin incorrectly use rubbing alcohol as an astringent, in the mistaken belief that the "sting" that results indicates the strong oil removal their skin needs.

The truth is that pure rubbing alcohol is the worst choice any man with acne-prone skin can make. Not only does it remove oil from the skin; it also removes moisture, overdrying the skin and causing surface flaking and dead skin-cell buildup—the same buildup, you'll remember, that contributes to the formation of acne blemishes in the first place. Instead of helping your skin, you'll only add to its problems in the long run.

It's better to use an astringent that contains alcohol within its formula, but as a lesser ingredient. What you need is a combination of less-harsh drying ingredients plus antibacterial agents such as camphor and sulfur, along with a certain amount of water to maintain the skin's essential moisture balance. This is an astringent that does not sting the skin, but does an effective cleansing and rebalancing job. It is gentle enough to be reapplied in the afternoon to refresh the skin and remove so-called "late-day shine" caused by the buildup of excess oiliness.

- **If I have acne, do I need a moisturizer?** This depends on how widespread your breakouts are. If you are like many adult men, you have blemishes only in the T-zone (the forehead and nose area) with clear skin on your cheeks, and will need a light moisturizing lotion (not a cream) in this area. Acne does not negate the need for eye cream.

- **If I have acne, does shaving affect it?** A man with acne should subject his skin to the least trauma possible. This would mean not shaving if you can, but I understand for many men this is impossible, either due to their work worlds or the fact that they do not like themselves with a beard. A compromise that I have worked out with many of my male clients during the years: to shave very carefully during the week, and to take the weekends "off" from shaving when possible, giving the skin a rest from the nicks and cuts that can accidentally spread infection. (For more on shaving basics, see Chapter 5.)

ACNE: SEPARATING MYTHS FROM FACTS

Down through the ages, acne has become associated with a full range of erroneous skin information, many times with embarrassing results for those patients already the victims of an unattractive skin condition. Here are some very important distinctions to be made between the myths and the facts.

- **Eating junk food does not automatically cause acne.** Would that it were so simple; then all we'd need do to clear up everyone's skin would be to ban potato chips! What is true is that some foods do seem to aggravate some skin problems **in some people.** What continues to baffle scientists is which foods in which people. Despite numerous reports of acne being caused by individual foods ranging from sugar to dairy products to french fries to seafood (one researcher feels iodine in seafood is the culprit), it has been impossible to prove that any of these claims are true for large groups of patients.

One interesting new theory postulates a connection between the high acne rate in this country and our predilection for a diet high in saturated fat. Switching to an eating plan that is lower in fat, higher in fresh fruits and vegetables and complex carbohydrates may (and I emphasize **may**) turn out to be as beneficial for your acne as it is for your heart.

What is clear is that the diet and acne connection seems to be a very individual one. Taking a dietary history of each patient is important to a skin care expert so that he or she can check for any pattern that may turn out to be a cause. Making changes in diet in an attempt to clear up the skin is a trial-and-error method, and must be viewed as only a part of a total skin-care routine. What is essential to understand is the overall link between total body health and good nutrition (see Chapter 7).

- **Stress causes acne.** This **may** be true, if you are suddenly under increased stress **and** you have a skin chemistry that is already prone to acne. The irony is that stress can just as readily cause overly dry skin as it can an overly oily or acne-prone complexion. What determines the difference is not different kinds of stress but different skin types! (For a full discussion of stress and relaxation, see Chapter 8.)

- **Too much sex causes acne; so does too little.** One look at these two contradictory statements should indicate their reliability! Acne does seem to be connected with the sex **hormones** in some way, but it has never been shown to have any connection whatsoever with the amount or lack of sexual activity or desire in a man's life. And acne is in no way a punishment for evil sexual thoughts or actions.

- **Oily skin causes acne.** This statement is either totally true or false. Every man with oily skin will not develop acne blemishes, but for those men who do, skin oiliness is often an accompanying problem.

If your skin is acne-prone, avoid the use of heavy skin creams or lotions, as well as the use of heavy gels, styling mousse or creams on your hair or scalp, which often seep down onto the surrounding forehead area and clog the pores, causing additional blemishes. Do change your pillowcases regularly, as skin oils that accumulate during the night can recontaminate the skin. Be aware that perspiration contains skin-irritating oils and bacteria, and should always be cleansed off the skin as soon as possible. The irritating potential of perspiration can easily be seen in the high prevalence of acne of the chest and shoulders in high school football players, who frequently perspire underneath their heavy shoulderpads. (For more on exercise and skin, see Chapter 9.)

- **Acne develops only on the face.** Nothing could be further from the truth. The chest and back are also common acne sites, particularly in adult-onset acne, and particularly for men. Treatments are basically the same as for facial acne, although at-home care must be even gentler, as the chest and back areas scar even more easily and less forgivingly than the face. Once severe scarring is present in these body areas, there is little that can be done to rid a patient of the scars. For this reason, I encourage any man who experiences breakouts in these areas to seek professional skin care advice as soon as possible.

- **Acne always causes scarring.** This, too, need not be true. While severe cystic acne is likely to leave the skin with some degree of scarring, much post-breakout pockmarking of the skin is the result not of the blemishes themselves, but of overzealous picking or squeezing of the skin either by a man himself or a less-than-qualified skin care practitioner. Never attempt to clean out a blemish yourself, and be aware that, although your skin may be somewhat red or slightly sensitive when you leave a skin care salon, no treatment should be painful when it is being done, and your skin should not be angrily inflamed by the treatments you receive. If you feel that your skin is being overmanipulated during a facial, say so. Remember that it is your skin that will bear the marks of mistreatment, and that you are entitled to and should be encouraged to ask as many questions about the treatment as you choose.

- **The sun is a great way to clear up acne.** While it may be true that, in very small doses, the ultraviolet rays of the sun do act to dry up acne blemishes, it may simply be the "masking" effect a bit of a tan can have on the breakouts. Skin that has a slightly red or tanned coloration simply looks less obviously inflamed than whiter, paler complexions. Too much sun can have a backfire effect on an acne-prone complexion. The reason: every suntan eventually begins to peel, at which point it is only natural for a man to apply an after-sun moisturizer or bronzing lotion to attempt to "extend" the tan. This adds to the buildup of oil and dead skin cells on his face, which become almost glued to the skin, and encourages the formation of additional skin blemishes.

The sun is also not without its own long-term skin hazards; no one wants to trade a bit of skin surface drying for the eventual proliferation of skin wrinkles and aging later on, let alone for the long-term increased risk of skin cancer (see Chapter 6).

I advise my acne-prone clients to enjoy the sun in moderation. Always use oil-free sunscreens and avoid overly creamy after-sun moisturizers. Always follow your tanning periods with a thorough professional facial, to discourage the buildup of dead skin cells on the skin surface and encourage the maintenance of healthy-looking skin. Too many acne patients make the mistake of skipping facials during the summer months, because they think their skin is improving, when in fact more damage than ever is going on beneath the skin surface.

BENZOYL PEROXIDE:
SKIN HELP OR HINDRANCE?

Many clients ask me about the over-the-counter anti-acne preparations sold in drugstores and supermarkets that contain varying concentrations of benzoyl peroxide. Are these a good place to begin self-treatment if you can't make it to a skin care salon? Yes and no, say many experts. While benzoyl peroxide does help to dry up acne lesions, it has become apparent that a good number of individuals do not tolerate the harshness of the ingredient very well. Benzoyl peroxide lotions and creams can cause skin irritation ranging from simple redness to severe dryness and itching and even, in some cases, allergic reaction. If you experience any adverse reaction, immediately discontinue use of such a product.

Never use these products around the eyes or on the mouth or neck, as these areas seem particularly prone to irritation. Do a patch test before using the product, applying it to a small area of your forearm, waiting 24 hours, and checking to see whether a reaction occurs.

Other topical preparations containing resorcinol or sulfur seem to be effective in healing existing lesions, note many experts, and are less likely to cause skin irritation of their own.

STRONGER STUFF: WHAT THE DOCTOR PRESCRIBES

Depending on the severity of your acne condition, dermatologists may prescribe any of the following drugs:

- **Oral antibiotics** including tetracycline and, less commonly, erythromycin, are thought to work primarily by reducing the number of P. acne bacteria growing within the follicle openings. Some patients develop stomach problems after several months on these drugs; other patients experience no side effects. Yeast infections are a not-uncommon side effect for women, but not for men.

- **Topical antibiotics** such as tetracycline or clindamycin are becoming increasingly common in use, as they allow a physician to target the treatment more directly at acne lesions and eliminate much of the risk of side effects. Available in liquid lotion form, these are applied on a daily basis (once or twice a day) by the patient, always using a fresh, clean cotton swab to avoid the spread of bacteria or infection.

- **Anti-inflammatory injections** of cortisone derivatives are sometimes used to hasten healing of large, severely inflamed cysts. These injections may be used directly into the cyst itself to concentrate the effect in one particular area or may be more generalized.

- **Accutane,** a drug that is a vitamin-A derivative, received FDA-approval for use only on severe, chronic cystic acne in 1983. It has proven to be surprisingly successful in clearing up acne lesions that were so severe that they failed to respond to various combinations of all of the above treatments. Some patients on the drug during its early testing have remained free of further acne lesions for as long as six years following initial treatment, during which time they have received no other medication.

Accutane is not without its side effects, ranging from dry mucous membranes (the lips and the inside of the nose in particular) to conjunctivitis, dry, itchy eyes, joint or muscle pain, slight hair loss, and elevation of blood triglyceride (fatty acid) levels. It cannot be given to women who are pregnant or who are planning on becoming pregnant during the course of treatment, and many physicians now request female patients get pregnancy tests as a precursor to prescribing the drug. All side effects, however, disappear with discontinuance of the drug, and there have been no reported ill effects on male reproductive organs at all.

• **In the future,** researchers hope to have more drugs that mimic Accutane's success without its side effects. Scientists also hope to gain a better, fuller understanding of the causes of acne so that it can become a skin concern of the past, and all of us can enjoy the pleasures of being blemish-free at every age.

CHAPTER FIVE

NO-FAULT SHAVING: HOW TO START THE DAY OFF RIGHT

"If you got it baby, flaunt it."

—the byword of the seventies
in America, attributed to
Mel Brooks

S having. For most men, it's the one skin routine they begin in their teens and continue for the rest of their lives. A young man's first shave is often fraught with high emotion. A sign of his proven manhood, it also brings on the fear of nicks and cuts, the jibes of friends who started shaving a little earlier, who tease, "what hairs have you got to shave off?" By the time men have reached their thirties, though, said one man in my salon, "shaving becomes one of those things you do automatically, like brushing your teeth, only it's more of a 'necessary evil' of being well-groomed!"

From a skin care point of view, this ambivalence is understandable. Shaving, it turns out, can be a man's skin's best friend or its worst enemy. What makes the difference are the shaving technique and products you use. To give you an idea of just "how much" shaving you do in your life, consider these facts: The average man has about 16,000 hairs on his face. In 55 years of shaving, he will remove literally 2½ feet of hair. Shaving not only separates the men from the boys, it also makes for the main difference between men's and women's skin.

SHAVING PLUSSES: YOUNGER-LOOKING SKIN

Shaving not only removes unwanted hairs from your face, it also lifts off dead skin cells, encouraging the exfoliation (or skin deflaking) that is the key to smooth, younger-looking skin. What we think of as "healthy" skin is skin that is translucent and even-surfaced, readily reflecting light. Shaving—when done correctly—helps keep skin free of the "debris" that can dull its appearance.

Every man has his own shaving style. One 40-year-old man told me that "you can probably tell more about a man's personality by watching him shave than by any other activity." There are the meticulous shavers who coat every inch of skin with a preshave preparation, then painstakingly remove every hair from their faces, rechecking each segment of skin before progressing to the next. Or the daredevil shaver, who brandishes his razor in a flourish of strokes like a medieval swordsman, come what may (which is, more often than not, nicks or cuts, plus a few strategic areas of less-than-perfectly shaved skin). Some men show themselves—and their mirrors—how tough they are through their shaving techniques; others exhibit an artistic sculptural gentleness in their shaving approach. Whatever attitude you choose, I am not out to change it. What I am concerned about, though, is that you protect your skin from what, if done incorrectly, can be needlessly harsh to your skin.

Just as the skin exfoliation of shaving can help your skin stay young, it can also, if done too roughly, cause excessive skin dryness and irritation. You can unknowingly remove skin cells that are not ready to be removed, or aggravate overdry already-flaking skin. What will help "smooth" the way for your shaving process and your skin are the products you use, the key to both a better shave and to less skin irritation in the long run.

STRAIGHT RAZOR OR ELECTRIC?

The choice here is a matter of personal preference. An electric shaver works by clipping off hairs; a razor slices hairs away. While some men swear by old-fashioned razors, others make equally loud claims for the superiority of electric shavers. Even fathers and sons disagree! Whatever method you choose, remember to use pre- and post-shave preparations formulated for that specific method.

GETTING THE BEST SHAVE:
A STEP-BY-STEP GUIDE

The first and most important step to no-fault shaving is this: Don't rush. It takes about five minutes to give yourself a safe, close shave. Cutting a minute off your time won't win you any medals—unless you consider battle scars desirable! Anyway, don't you think you're worth spending five minutes on in the morning? I do—and I'm certain you'll agree once you see how no-fault shaving makes for a smoother, closer, more comfortable shave.

Before you begin, take a minute to examine your face and neck in a magnifying mirror. Note the direction in which your hair grows. Whether you choose to shave with or against your natural hair growth pattern is a matter

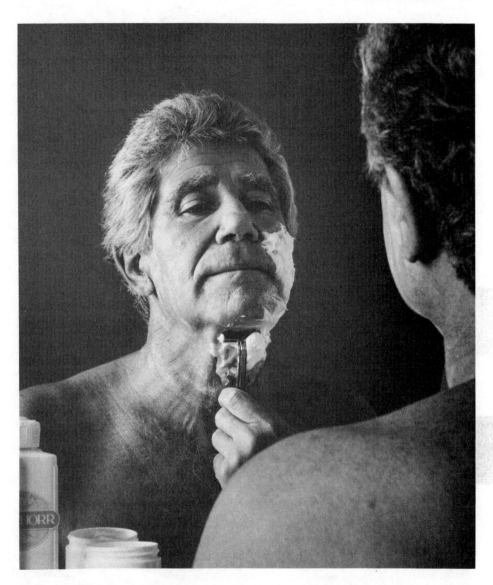

The most difficult area to shave: the neck.

of personal choice; most men usually adopt one method and stick with it. One area where problems sometimes occur is on the neck, where hair can grow in several different directions. If you have this tendency, you may find that shaving in different directions (as long as you never go over the same area more than twice) makes for the smoothest and least irritating shave.

If you use a straight razor, follow these steps:

- Begin with clean equipment—your razor **and** your hands.
- Cleanse your face with a cleansing lotion appropriate to your skin type.

- Splash warm water on your face to open pores and soften beard hairs. (To achieve a thorough softening effect, many men like to shave after a shower or bath—an especially good idea if you have a tough beard or sensitive skin.)
- Apply a gentle wash-off cream (a pre-shave softener) to further soften beard; rinse off after 3 to 4 minutes. (If your skin is highly sensitive, you may want to substitute a moisturizer to be left on your skin.)
- Apply shaving foam, cream, or gel and wait 2 minutes before you begin to shave to "set up" your beard. (A word of skin expertise here: Despite the fact that about 75 percent of shaving cream buyers choose an aerosol product, I feel that creams or gels are better choices because they are worked into the face with the gentle stimulation of the fingers, and provide better skin and beard coverage, more skin-softening effectiveness than a product that is simply sprayed onto the skin surface.)
- Begin shaving the upper cheeks, then work down to the lower right and left sides of the face and the upper lip. Then shave the chin and, finally, the neck. By thinking of your face in terms of four quadrants, and beginning with the areas where the hair is sparsest and finishing where hair is denser and thicker, you expose the "toughest" beard area to the softening benefits of your pre-shave product longest and get the smoothest possible shave.
- Rinse face with lukewarm water. Pat (don't rub) dry.
- Apply a gentle, nonalcohol after-shave cream or lotion-formula balm (see below) followed by a moisturizer.

If you use an electric shaver, follow these steps:

- Remember, the drier the skin the better.
- Keep your shaver clean with the specially-provided small brush. This will not only give you a closer shave, but will help to reduce skin irritation.
- Use a soothing after-shave balm plus a moisturizer after every shave.

POST-SHAVING SMARTS: TO BURN IS NOT BETTER

Men, being the tough-minded sex, have somehow been convinced that the more an after-shave lotion burns, the better it "works." Nothing could be further from the truth. The purpose of an after-shave product is not to kill bacteria but to soothe and "calm" a man's skin. It should feel refreshing, yes, but not burning. And it should not be high in alcohol content (as most fragranced liquids are), as this will only add to any post-shave skin dryness or irritation.

The best choices are after-shave balms, available in lotion, cream, or gel versions, often in fragranced or non-fragranced options. If your skin tends to be very dry, you'll probably want to boost the soothing effects with a rich moisturizing cream; if you have combination or oily skin, a lighter moisturizer is a good choice. Whatever your skin type, don't overlook your neck, which deserves the soothing benefits as well!

SPECIAL SHAVING TIPS

This advice is culled from my male clients and from my years of experience in the skin care field to help every man get the best shave possible:

- To minimize irritation and lessen the chances of developing ingrown hairs (more on these later), don't shave over any one skin area more than twice. Don't worry about any stray hairs; no one will be examining your skin with a magnifying lens.

- Don't use a dull blade; you'll get less of a shave, more skin redness and irritation.

- Try to shave only once a day. If you get a heavy 5 o'clock shadow and feel you must shave again before going out for the evening, use an electric shaver rather than a blade for less chance of irritation.

- One trick that helps some men lessen the "brutality" of daily shaving is to alternate between an electric shaver and a straight-edge razor.

- Many men find that giving their skin a "mini-vacation" from shaving by taking the weekend off and letting their skin feel free helps to heal red or irritated areas, make for smoother, easier shaves the rest of the week. Others even grow a beard for a month or so once every year, then resume shaving again. Who knows, you may even find that you like your bearded "look" and want to keep it for a while.

- For a quick nick or cut repair, dab on a spot of mud-based face masque. It will help "tighten" pores and encourage blood to clot. (Don't use talc on your face as it tends to clog pores and encourage breakouts.)

- Don't shave right before exercise, as perspiring on newly-shaved skin can be especially irritating. Perspiration is highly alkaline and can exacerbate skin flaking and dryness. Wait until after your post-workout shower to shave.

- If you have acne-prone skin, be especially careful when shaving. Ideally, it's best not to shave in areas where skin is already broken out. If accidental cuts do occur in areas where skin infection is present, be certain to recleanse the area and apply your usual topical anti-acne preparation.

- Extremely dry or capillary-prone skin can also increase a man's shaving sensitivity. Be certain to use preshave skin softening products suited to your skin type; choose rich moisturizing formulas low in alcohol for post-shave use.

- Never shave dry when using a straight razor. Hair has the hardness of copper wire when it's a stubble and requires excessive pressure to be removed, even with a fresh blade.

COPING WITH INGROWN HAIRS

Ingrown hairs (or pseudofolliculitis) are most common among men with coarse or curly hair; they can be unattractive and, in many cases, even painful. Shaving with the proper products and technique can help to minimize the problem, and there are certain things a man can do at home to remove isolated ingrown hairs.

An ingrown hair is basically a hair that grows back in on itself, repenetrating the skin. Once it comes back into the skin, it is attacked by the body's natural defenses, just as any foreign body is, setting up the stage for later, painful infection. Black men, whose hair tends to be curly, are most prone to the problem. Ironically, the closer you shave, the more you may encourage ingrown hairs, as only short hairs can reenter the skin once they've come out.

You can remove one or two ingrown hairs yourself with the help of a fine needle and tweezers sterilized in boiling water. Gently try to "flick out" the hair with the needle, then to pull it out with the tweezer. If you don't succeed in two attempts, give up. Trying any further will only cause the removal of skin, which will leave a scar that may be even more unsightly. Always remove ingrown hairs at night, and follow with the application of a medicated drying lotion to give skin a chance to recover overnight. Difficult-to-remove hairs may need professional help from a dermatologist or skin-care expert or, in recurrent cases, from an electrologist.

If ingrown hairs are a recurrent problem and you've developed unsightly "razor bumps," what can you do? New medical studies show that electrolysis—permanent hair removal done by a professionally-trained practitioner—may be the answer. The source of this new information is a dermatologist, who was consulted by the Air Force to help them solve the problems of black servicemen whose recurrent bouts with ingrown hairs prevented them from meeting the Air Force's clean-shaven requirement. This doctor found that electrolysis—the one proven method of permanent hair removal—could be successful in the destruction of ingrown hairs at their "roots." What worked in this one study was the insulated bulbous (IB) probe electrolysis machine, which could be gently curved into the follicle opening to treat distorted or curly hairs.

To be successful, electrolysis requires repeated treatments. At your first visit with a specialist, he or she will be able to tell you roughly how many treatments will be needed and how long each session will be, as well as the approximate total cost. A good way to find a qualified electrolygist is through a skin care expert or dermatologist who has treated you in the past. (For more on referrals, see page 177.)

POSITIVE REINFORCERS: AT-HOME DELIGHTS

To provide a welcome change of pace from commercial products, try these three simple at-home skin whip-ups, fine for every skin type.

Cucumber Cleansing Lotion

Blend together ½ cup strained cucumbers and ¼ cup milk. Apply to face with cotton. Let it absorb into the skin. Don't rinse off. Ideal for morning and evening use or for a quick midday skin refresher.

Strawberry After-Shave Mask

Mash 2 strawberries. Mix together with 1 teaspoon sour cream. Apply to face and leave on for 10 minutes. Use twice a week.

Peppermint After-Shave Lotion

Mix 2 ounces of witch hazel extract with 2 ounces of peppermint oil (or lemon oil if you prefer). Apply to face after each shave; follow up with a moisturizer appropriate to your skin type.

CHAPTER SIX

SUN AND SKIN: PLAYING IT SAFE

> The French are true romantics. They feel the only difference between a man of 40 and one of 70 is 30 years of experience.
>
> —Maurice Chevalier

If you're like most American men, chances are that as soon as the calendar turns over to May, you start thinking about your summer tan. After all, most men think they look healthier, wealthier, and sexier with a bit of brown in their complexions. Most men too, love spending their summer weekends outdoors, be it lounging on the beach, playing with their kids in the pool, or going for a leisurely sail or a "serious" fishing trip. In a world where most of us spend our working hours cooped up in an office, a factory, or a store, time spent outside basking in the sun is the ultimate luxury.

Yet the notion of a "healthy-looking" suntan is a complete misnomer. The same rays of the sun that lift our spirits, warm our bodies, and bring a blush of pink to our cheeks also work to rob us of our looks and our health. Simply put, the ultraviolet rays of the sun are our skin's worst enemies. They cause the skin to wrinkle, to sag, to become freckled and discolored, to look dry and leathery. In the long run, sun exposure is the single biggest cause of skin aging—and it is also the prime culprit in most cases of skin cancer.

As a report from The Dermatology Foundation notes, skin cancer increases in incidence the closer the population lives to the equator; those who are of fair skin with light eyes are the most vulnerable. Reduced sun exposure will reduce the risk of skin cancer. The attractiveness of having a tan must be balanced with the awareness that the deeper your tan is now, the sooner you will get wrinkles in the future.

The good news is that it is never too late to protect your skin from the sun—and there are safe ways to get a tan, thanks to the new science of sunscreens. What's more, studies now reveal that the skin repairs itself over time, so even a man who spent all of his teen years and twenties basking in the sun each summer can save his skin by starting to protect it in his thirties.

My own experience with the sun illustrates both the damage it can do and the skin's miraculous ability to recover. Growing up in Israel and living on a kibbutz in the desert from the age of 12 to 19, I was totally carefree and

65

never gave a thought to skin care or protecting my skin from the elements. The harsh desert sun was already quite strong by the time we began work in the fields at 6 A.M., and I was always freckled and bronzed. By the time I was 20, I had the brown, leathery skin of a woman at least twice my age. When I came to the United States and became involved in the skin care profession, I learned how bad the sun was for my skin and stopped baking myself each summer. Within a few years, my freckles had lessened, my skin had become softer and smoother, and I looked younger than I had at 20. These days, I stay out of the sun during the heat of the noon hours, and always wear a sunscreen whenever I am outdoors. My skin looks younger and clearer now than when I look at pictures of myself twenty years ago!

SMART SUNNING

Dermatologists note that sun exposure is not simply a matter of lying on the beach, but of playing tennis, going to the ball game, walking to and from the office and a lunch appointment. Men who are regularly exposed to the sun should use a light, lotion-based sunscreen as an after-shave balm. The throat, chest, ears, and the backs of the hands (where age spots often first appear) should all be protected—as should the top of a bald head. Look for a product that contains PABA (para-amino-benzoic acid), PABA esters, zinc oxide, or titanium oxide.

Since it takes a while for a sunscreen to sink into the skin, it's best to put one on 15 to 30 minutes before going outdoors. It also makes sense to stay out of the sun between 10 A.M. and 2 P.M., when two-thirds of the day's ultraviolet rays reach the earth.

How to Choose a Sunscreen

You need to know your SPFs (the abbreviation for Sun Protection Factor, which most companies now use to label their sun products). The SPF ratings range from 2 to 15 (usually 2, 4, 6, 8, 10, or 15). The number indicates the strength of the suscreen: how much longer you can stay in the sun with it than without it and not get burned. While sunscreens protect you from much of the sun's damage, they do not prevent you from getting a tan. The tan you get with a sunscreen will often take longer to achieve, but it will also be a longer-lasting tan, and be less likely to peel unattractively as sunburn often does.

A product with an SPF of 2, for example, will allow you to stay in the sun twice as long as you could otherwise. Two is the lowest SPF—typical of "dark-tanning oils"—and offers minimal protection. If you are someone who burns easily, wearing an SPF of 2 is not going to help you; you will simply get a bad burn in 10 minutes rather than 5!

The SPF you need depends on two basic factors: how easily you burn and how much sun exposure you have had already. A suntan offers some

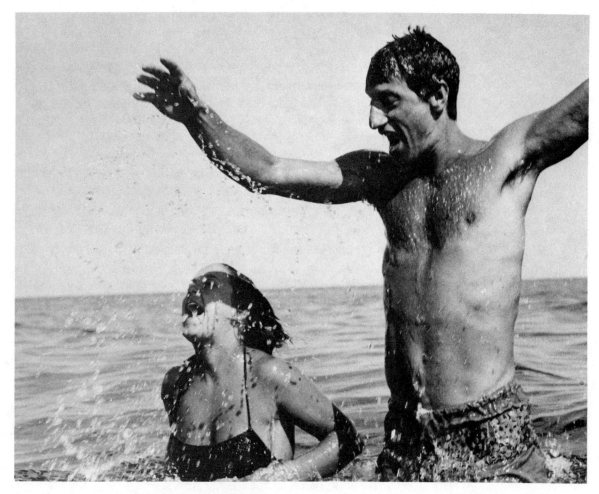

Key to skin safety outdoors: protective sunscreens.

(although not that much) protection against burning ultraviolet rays. Contrary to popular belief, having dark or black skin does not make you immune to sun damage. It may take the sun longer to wreak havoc on your skin, but you won't totally be able to avoid its ill effects.

The critical point in choosing your SPF is to use a stronger one during the first few days you're in the sun. Most men do the opposite, trying to get as much sun as possible in the first few days at the beach or on vacation. Yet the first two to three days are the time when you can get badly sunburned because you have no protection; it takes the body a few days to build up its natural defense of added pigment (or melanin) in the skin. Even if you don't begin to look tan for a while, don't let that lull you into thinking you are not getting any sun; rushing things will probably just result in a bad burn.

To take full advantage of the sun and protect your skin while still getting some color, you may need more than one sunscreen product. Use one with a higher SPF for the first week or so until a slight tan builds up; then use another with a lower SPF to protect slightly-tanned skin while allowing it to darken further. Your collection should also include a complete sunblock (SPF 15), which will be needed when you plan on spending the whole day outdoors or when sailing (more on water plus sun later).

In general, the following SPF strengths work best for the six skin types doctors have identified (NOTE: Always switch to a higher SPF in tropical sunshine, when close to the equator):

- TYPE I—always burns easily, never tans—SPF 10 or 15 (don't even try to tan; your skin will simply not adapt a brown color)
- TYPE II—always burns easily, tans minimally—SPF 10, then 8 once you have been out in the sun a week or longer.
- TYPE III—burns moderately, tans slowly to light brown—SPF 8, then 6.
- TYPE IV—burns minimally, always tans well- to medium brown—SPF 8, then 6.
- TYPE V—rarely burns, tans to dark brown—SPF 6 to cut down on ultraviolet exposure.
- TYPE VI—never burns, deeply pigmented naturally—SPF 6 to cut down on ultraviolet exposure.

What about SPF's 4 and 2? I don't believe in them, unless you use them in the spring or fall when the sun is less intense. In the heat of summer, they simply do not provide enough protection against the aging effects of the sun; use them as a moisturizer if you wish on an everyday basis, but do not rely on them as true protection in the hot summer sun. One day, I hope, the FDA will sanction an SPF number 30, for real sun protection!

BEYOND SPFs: APPLICATION IS KEY

It's important to reapply your sunscreen often and to take breaks from the sun to allow your skin to recover and your body to refresh itself as well.

I no longer advise any man, no matter what his skin type, to lie in the sun for hours on end. If you insist on basking in the sun, do so for no more than 20 minutes at a time. Then get up and go into the shade for 10 minutes, rinse your face with cool water, apply a moisturizer, then reapply your sunscreen. Drink a cool glass of water; the heat and sun are dehydrating and your body needs to replace its fluids.

It's important to reapply sunscreen during the day, especially if you perspire heavily or go in and out of the water. Many of the newest sunscreens are waterproof or water-resistant; this means they will provide some protection while you are swimming, but it does not mean they will not rub off when you come out and dry yourself with a towel. Always be certain to reapply sunscreen before you go swimming; in clear water, 90 to 95 percent of the ultraviolet rays that hit the surface can reach your skin even if you're swimming or snorkeling three feet under! Read the label to see how often your brand of sunscreen needs to be reapplied.

DANGER ZONES:
EYES, LIPS, EARS

How you apply your sunscreen will help determine not only how even your tan is, but also how much of your face and body you have prevented from damage. Don't forget the sensitive skin of the nose, the ears, the shoulders, and—if you don't have a full head of hair—the top of your head; the sun beats down on us from above and those are the first spots it hits.

The lips are also sensitive to sun damage; look for a lip balm that contains a sunscreen and reapply it often. Be aware of the delicate skin area between the lips and the nose, where unwary sun worshippers often get a painful burn.

The eyes need double protection; not only is this the most sun-sensitive, vulnerable skin, but the eyes themselves are susceptible to damage from ultraviolet rays. Look for new sunglasses that not only shield you from the sun's glare but also offer protection from ultraviolet rays. When in the sun for long periods of time, put cold compresses on your eyes to avoid the puffiness that often follows a day at the seashore. When sailing, wear a big hat plus sunglasses; the glare of the sun off the water is as damaging to your eyes as it is to your skin.

MODERATION:
KEY TO LOOKING GOOD FOREVER

If you've been reading all my warnings so far, your thoughts may be roving to images of a man swathed in hat, beach robe, earmuffs and layers of sun products seeking to live the good life. What fun is going to the beach, you may be asking, if you couldn't play volleyball or go for a jog along the shore without worrying every minute about your skin? I am not saying that you must forsake outdoor activities and become a hermit in the summertime;

what I am saying is that once you understand the damage, the dryness, the wrinkling, and the aging that can come from sun exposure, you will want to make sun protection a regular habit, and you will learn to be moderate in your pursuit of a tan.

One of my clients told me an interesting story that offers some insight into wise suntanning. He had always gone to the beach every summer, as most New Yorkers do, braving the traffic out to the Hamptons every Friday night and back into the city on Sunday evening every weekend all summer long. He loved the sun, was brown as a berry by early July, and continued to bake his skin through to the last rays of September. Suddenly, on his thirty-fifth birthday, he looked in the mirror and as he said, "I saw a man who looked 50 staring back at me, with leathery skin, wrinkling around my lips and eyes, and a tired-out look. I knew I needed help for my skin **now.**" He came to me and I told him the truth: What he was seeing reflected in the mirror were the cumulative effects of years of sun damage, the effects that often don't show up for years afterward. I convinced him that he had to start protecting his skin now, that there was little that he could do to repair the wrinkling, but that time is often a good skin healer. He began using sunscreens (SPF 15) regularly and now, years later, he tells me that he looks better than ever. His skin is smoother, more richly moisturized, and some of the leathery feel has been replaced with fresher, smoother skin. "What is amazing," he tells me, "is that I always thought sun protection meant living an indoor life, but I still play sports, go swimming, enjoy the beach, and still protect my skin. I get a nice bronzed look by late summer but it is a healthy looking bronze, not a tanned leather look like I used to get. When I look at old photos of myself during the summer, I wonder why I ever thought that dark, dark tan was attractive."

SPECIAL PRECAUTIONS:
SKIN AND HEALTH GUARDS

- Avoid using perfume or cologne or highly scented aftershave when you're in the sun; any spot you dab it on may be sensitive to the sun. Likewise, avoid shaving right before or after sun exposure; the sensitiviy of your skin will be magnified.

- Certain kinds of medications can cause the skin to have a photosensitive reaction—even a few minutes in the sun can cause an extreme burn or rash. Check first with your doctor, especially if you are being treated for acne, keratoses, diabetes or high blood pressure, or are taking antibiotics, tranquilizers, or diuretics.

- Be aware that the higher the altitude, the closer you are to the sun, and the more intense its effects will be. In the mountains in the summer, the air may feel cool but the sun will be quite strong as there is less air (and pollution) to filter the ultraviolet rays. Skiers are especially prone to severe sunburns and need to be careful in applying sunscreens and rich moisturizers to guard against burning and moisture loss.

- Sunning, swimming, and the outdoor life can also take their toll on your hair. One of the easiest ways to shield your hair from the sun is to cover it with a breathable cotton weave or straw hat. An alternative is to use one of the new sunscreen-containing products meant especially for the hair. Look for setting gels and mousses as well as creamy conditioners that can be applied to hair before sun exposure, protect the hair from ultraviolet rays and the drying effects of chlorine and salt water. Never allow your hair to dry in the sun after a swim without rinsing it with clear water, since sunlight plus chlorine or salt water combine to cause dry, brittle hair and split ends. If you're heading for a beach where fresh water won't be handy, tuck a thermos of club soda or mineral water into your beachbag for a refreshing, bubbly rinse—and a healthful drink as well.

- Watch what you eat in the heat of summer. Heavy or greasy foods can cause upset stomachs. What your body needs most is water; so drink plenty of it, plus eat water-rich foods like fresh fruits, melon, apples, and vegetables. While many men love to drink beer at the beach, this is not the best choice; beer is not only fattening, but, like any alcoholic beverage, it actually robs the body of water rather than supplementing the cells' fluid needs. Opt for fresh-squeezed orange juice, lemonade without sugar, club soda, or mineral water instead. Salty snacks will make you thirstier, so choose a frozen yogurt, a tall glass of iced tea, or a cold platter of fresh vegetables.

- Don't head for the sauna or the steam room immediately after being out in the sun. Your skin will already be overheated; adding more warmth can intensify a sunburn or even bring one on, if it hasn't yet surfaced. Save the sauna for the day after, when you'll want to take a day off from sunning.

- Remember that the water—in a pool, in the ocean, when sailing or boating—acts as a mirror, intensifying the ability of the sun to heat and burn your skin. If you'll be spending a good deal of time near the water, switch to a higher SPF than usual and keep reapplying it. Even men who say they never burn often are taken by surprise when they spend a day on a boat, being cooled by the sea breezes, and come out of the shower in the evening with an incredibly bright red sunburn. A man with fair skin should wear long-sleeved shirts, long pants and a hat on a boat, if he doesn't want to be heading into the cabin after an hour in the sun!

- Don't let the sun catch you by surprise. I can't tell you how many of my clients have gotten sunburned when riding in a convertible with the top down, or simply driving with one arm bent out an open window. Riding your bicycle to the grocery store is great exercise, but it is also time that your skin is bared to the sun, so use a sunscreen. Eating lunch outdoors on a warm summer day is certainly relaxing, but count that hour into your weekly sun "quotient" and be aware that a sunburn is one thing that most of us never plan for—and that our skin suffers for, in the long run.

- You can never be too young or too old to suffer sun damage. If you have children, teach them the sun protection habit when young; they'll thank you for it when they're older. Likewise, you never "outgrow" the need for sun protection; there's no such thing as being too old to be attractive.

- **Never** use a reflector—it is equivalent to baking yourself in the oven! Never go out in the sun with baby oil or coconut oil slathered on your skin; it would be like turning your body into a French fry.

- While clouds seem to mask the sun, they only block the light, **not** the ultraviolet rays. You can get a worse burn on a cloudy day than a clear, sunny one, because you will be lulled into not feeling the sun on your skin. Apply a sunscreen whatever the weather whenever you're spending time outdoors in summer.

- Some people develop an allergy to PABA (paraaminobenzoic acid), the main ingredient in most sunscreens. If you do, look for one of the new PABA-free formulas (ask your pharmacist if you are uncertain).

- If your skin tends to be oily, avoid greasy or heavy sun creams as these can block pores and encourage blemishes. Instead, choose a light lotion formula (some are even labeled "for oily skin"). If your skin is very dry, you may want to apply a light moisturizer over your sunscreen for additional protection.

In short, while tanning may be part of the American way, avoiding intense sun exposure is the only way to ensure that your skin will be given a fair chance as it moves through time's natural processes. Whatever your ethnic background, be aware that the skin remembers. Although fair-skinned individuals may "show" sun bathing sooner, every skin type is vulnerable.

Each exposure to ultraviolet rays takes its toll. In most cases, it takes years for the damage to become visible, when it is often too late to correct.

IF YOU'VE OVERDONE IT: SUNBURN RELIEF

Sun puts the skin on the defensive; tanning is a retaliation process, the marshalling of the skin's melanocytes (or pigment-producing cells) to protect the underlayers of the skin from the harmful rays of the sun. Light-skinned individuals have far less melanin (or pigment) producing potential than those with olive or black skin. Whatever your skin type, too much sun can equal sunburn, comparable to the effect of sticking your hand into a too-hot oven. Even black skin can get burned, although the darker your complexion, the longer it will take.

While a sunburn is most obvious—and uncomfortable—on the skin's outer layers, it is also a reflection of damage under the skin's surface. Sunburn indicates a breaking down of the skin's connective fibers, the type of damage that eventually leads to wrinkled, sagging skin. A sunburn, in other words, is the augury of aging skin to come.

A severe sunburn, as any other major burn, can be painful—and at its most severe form can land you in the hospital. The best thing to do for a mild sunburn is to cool your skin with a soak in a lukewarm (not hot) bath, with three teaspoons of baking soda mixed in for added skin-soothing. If the skin is inflamed, you may want to take two aspirins for their anti-inflammatory effect. Compresses soaked in cool water, milk, or iced tea can soothe burned facial skin or puffy eyelids. While some people opt for anesthetic sprays or lotions sold in drugstores, it is not uncommon to develop an allergic reaction to these.

If your skin feels hot to the touch, apply a head-to-toe plain yogurt masque, leave on for ten minutes, then shower off with cool water. Avoid rubbing your skin with a loofah, washcloth, or a towel, as this will increase skin tenderness. Instead, pat skin dry and apply moisturizer (one with aloe, if possible, as this plant's extracts are natural burn-healers).

If your skin is peeling, apply a rich moisturizer to lessen surface flakiness, supplemented at night by a moisturizing mask. **Never** pull off about-to peel skin. The skin will fall off when it is ready; pulling it off too soon will reveal red, raw skin, and cause irritation. If your skin has become very dry, add three cups of whole milk to a lukewarm bath and let your body soak for 10 minutes.

Any blistering or highly painful sunburn should be brought to a physician's attention, **not** self-treated.

TANNING SALONS: DOUBLE DANGER

In the endless pursuit of having a year-round tan, more and more men have been visiting the tanning centers opening in health clubs and free-standing "salons." While their advertisements claim that these centers provide a "safe" tan, this is simply not so, according to a recent article in **The FDA Consumer** magazine. Any tan, whether acquired indoors or out, poses hazards to the skin; in some cases, a few minutes in a tanning center can be more dangerous than a full day at the beach.

Some tanning salons claim they are "safe" because they use only UVA radiation, as opposed to old-fashioned UVB, or "burning" rays. While it is true that the UVB ultraviolet rays will burn the skin faster than UVA, the newest scientific research shows that all types of ultraviolet light may be dangerous to the skin, and that UVA may be more harmful in the long run than UVB. The reason: UVA penetrates deeper into the skin than UVB, and may increase the risk of other health hazards such as edema [swelling], vascular system damage, and skin damage [such as premature aging of the skin, resulting in a wrinkled, leathery look]. It may also increase the chances of skin cancer, noted one recent report. Sunlamp, tanning booth or tanning bed—all are equally dangerous to a man's appearance and health.

As if skin aging and skin cancer hazards weren't reasons enough to avoid them, tanning salons are of concern for another reason, according to speakers at a recent conference sponsored by the American Academy of Dermatology. Because they are not licensed by any regulatory agencies, tanning salons are not checked by any outside inspectors for the amount or intensity of the radiation to which they expose their customers. Therefore, there is no way for a consumer to judge what a "safe" period, if there is any such thing, in such a salon could be. As one dermatologist recommended, "Avoid these centers if you care about the look and the health of your body and your skin."

WHY REAL MEN DON'T NEED SUNTANS

The true elite are those who look youngest longest and still manage to have a year-round healthy glow. These men have learned that real men don't bake in the sun; a little sun exposure, with the proper sunscreen, goes a long way. With a little "outside help"—i.e., one of the new skin bronzers—a man who gets a little bit of a tan, slowly, can look as if he got a lot more and still safeguard his skin from wrinkling and aging. To learn how to use a bronzer without looking as if you're wearing makeup—while looking as if you have a superb tan—turn to Chapter 11.

CHAPTER SEVEN

DIET
AND
NUTRITION

You don't live to eat;
you eat to live.

—adapted from Benjamin Franklin's
Poor Richard's Almanac

Whoever coined the phrase, "We are what we eat," knew what he or she was talking about. When it comes to the body's inner and outer health, few things are more essential than good nutrition. Diet affects everything from cell metabolism to the "fueling" of muscles to the healthy glow of skin. Well-balanced, deliciously nutritious meals are the body's interior insurance that the skin's inner needs are being fulfilled.

The most frequent complaint I hear from my male clients when I ask if they are eating a balanced diet is "Who has the time?" While it is true that our modern, urbanized lives mean that few of us grow our own vegetables, raise our own dairy cows or hunt or fish for this evening's supper, eating healthfully does not have to be time-consuming. One glance at the menus in even the finest restaurants will show you the new emphasis on lighter, more health-oriented dining—even New York City's Four Seasons restaurant now devotes a section of its menu to "Spa Cuisine!" Shopping at the supermarket offers healthy choices even for those men whose cooking abilities are nonexistent. There are frozen dinners that now contain less fat and salt than in the past, takeout meals based on satisfying a man's nutritional awareness along with his gourmet tastes. (Think, for example, of spinach pasta and fresh vegetables instead of fettucine alfredo smothered in cream sauce.) A balanced diet doesn't mean you have to give up Chinese, Italian, or Mexican restaurants. It does mean that your food choices will be wiser, but no less enjoyable.

BALANCING YOUR DIET:
WHAT IT MEANS

- **The first rule of healthful eating: put variety in your diet.** The human body needs about 40 different nutrients to stay healthy; no single

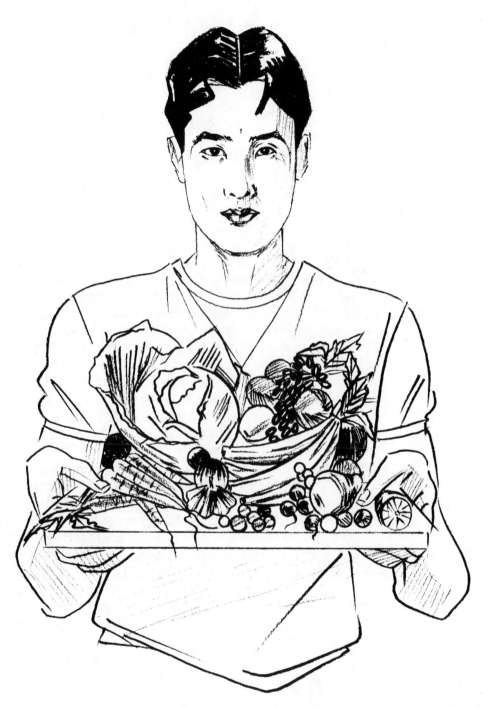

A balanced diet is wise skin insurance.

food can provide everything it needs. The greater the range of different foods you eat every day, the less likely you are to develop a deficiency or an excess of any single nutrient (and the less likely you are to be exposed to excessive amounts of any type of chemical contaminants in any single food item).

The simplest way to assure variety in your diet is by making selections from each of the major "food groups" daily:

- fruits and vegetables (four or more servings daily)
- cereals, whole grain and enriched breads, and grains such as rice or pasta (at least four servings daily)
- meats, poultry, eggs, fish

    or

    - dry peas and beans (soybeans, kidney beans, lima beans, black-eyed peas). These are all excellent sources of low-fat protein, especially when eaten in combination with whole grains and breads. (two servings daily)
    - milk, cheese, yogurt, dairy products (two servings daily)

Fruits and vegetables are excellent sources of vitamins C and A, note nutrition experts at the U.S. Department of Agriculture. Whole grain and enriched breads are prime sources of iron and B-vitamins, while meats not only supply protein and iron but also thiamine and vitamin B-12. Dairy products, essential sources of calcium and vitamin D, should be eaten in low-fat versions when possible.

- **Avoid overeating.** Being overweight is not only unattractive, it is dangerous to your health. Obesity increases a man's risk of high blood pressure, heart attack, and diabetes, note studies supported by the U.S. Department of Health, Education, and Welfare. And skin that is "stretched" to accommodate excess fat often becomes loose and saggy if you lose weight later in adulthood (more on this later).

The biggest problem many executives have is avoiding "expense account" stomach bulge. Here's the simplest way to control your eating habits: If you must dine out often for business, decide what you'll eat **before** you reach the restaurant (broiled fish of the day, broiled chicken, or steamed lobster; no fish in cream sauce, no creamy salad dressings—just a green salad with lemon juice and vinegar) and then simply ask the waiter for it. Don't hesitate to ask for half-portions, or to skip the soup and appetizer and just have a main course. Your business associates may urge you to eat more, but you know that deep down inside, they'll envy your personal control—

and may even take your self-discipline as further proof that they've chosen the right person to be doing business with!

If you do overeat at lunch, then scale down your dinner intake. One old, sensible adage advises to eat a king's breakfast, a peasant's lunch, and a beggar's dinner in order to maintain a slim physique—and this makes sense because we "use up" the most amount of food when we're most active, have little need for food before we're going to sleep. Learn to think of food in terms of daily eating, and to make mental trade-offs between several meals to keep your caloric intake in check.

While your doctor can best tell you the exact weight that's ideal for you, experts from the Department of Health, Education and Welfare found that the best weight for most adults is the one that their bodies chose naturally at the age of 20 to 25 (unless, of course, you were extremely overweight at that age). Their simple guidelines for improving your eating habits and maintaining a healthful weight range are: Learn to eat slowly, to prepare or request smaller portions, and to avoid "seconds" (even if your wife or mother sometimes confuses second helpings with proof of your love!).

• **Avoid too much fat and cholesterol.** Scientists have proven a correlation between the amount of fat (especially the animal fat cholesterol) in a man's diet and his risk not only of heart attack but of certain types of cancer as well. Cutting down on cholesterol doesn't mean you must become a vegetarian; it may simply be a matter, say, of eating red meat once or twice a week rather than three times, or having less mayonnaise in your tuna salad, substituting mustard or vinegar instead.

Some simple tips for cutting back on the fat in your diet:

1. Choose lean meat, fish, poultry, dry peas, and beans as your protein sources. Be aware that meat is "graded" by the amount of fat it contains, with "prime" steak the highest in fat of all!

2. When preparing meat, trim away all visible fat before **and** after cooking. Moderate your intake of eggs and liver.

3. Eat less high-fat butter, cream, hydrogenated margarines, shortenings, and coconut oil. Read labels to look for these hidden fat sources. Look instead for lighter, more healthful safflower, sunflower, or soybean oils.

• **Eat foods that provide adequate fiber.** The average American diet is relatively low in fiber, which is one reason so many of us suffer from digestive diseases. Eating more fiber is also among recommendations made in a recent report issued by the American Cancer Society which noted that "even if fiber itself may not prove to have a protective effect against cancer, high fiber-containing fruits, vegetables, and cereals can be recommended as a wholesome substitute for fatty foods." Fiber can help to fight constipation, diverticulosis, and some types of "irritable bowel syndrome." Allowing your body to cleanse itself naturally without the use of artificial laxatives can also help balance your skin's self-cleansing process, improving the texture and tone of your skin in the long run. There is also growing evidence that switching to a diet with greater amounts of natural fiber can decrease a man's risk of both adult-onset diabetes and cancer of the colon.

• **Avoid too much sugar and salt.** Studies indicate that the average American consumes as much as 130 pounds of sugar a year! Yet sugar, honey, jams and jellies are primarily "empty" calories, providing quick energy bursts followed by equally quick energy lows, giving the body no fuel to draw on as the day goes on.

What's more, sugar is a proven cause of dental decay. Besides cutting down on the sugar you add to your coffee or tea, there are other easy ways to decrease the sugar in your diet: Select fresh fruits rather than canned; plain breads and rolls rather than donuts or sticky buns; and be aware that the words sucrose, glucose, maltose, dextrose, lactose, or fructose on food labels all indicate sugar has been added during processing.

American men also tend to overuse the salt shaker, liberally salting food during and after cooking, often without even tasting it first! The major risk of all this salting is the development of high blood pressure, a problem affecting approximately 17 percent of adults in this country and one that continues to be on the rise.

Frequent sources of "hidden" salt are processed foods, ranging from canned vegetables to stuffing mixes to salty pretzels and corn chips. Even over-the-counter medications like antacids often contain surprisingly high levels of salt. Learn to read labels, and be aware that any chemical compound containing sodium has the potential to increase your blood pressure, as well as to increase your body's tendency to retain water and develop an unattractive "bloated" look.

FOOD:
YOUR BODY'S BUILDING BLOCKS

The human body has the unique capacity to repair and replenish itself from the inside out. Food not only gives us the energy to get through the demands of each day, but provides our bodies with the raw materials for this constant replenishing process. Following is a basic overview of food's role in maintaining a healthy, vibrant body.

Protein   One of the most important elements for the maintenance of good health and vitality, protein is the major source of "building materials" for muscles, blood, skin, hair, nails and internal body organs. During digestion the large molecules of proteins are decomposed into simpler units called amino acids; the body requires approximately 22 amino acids in a specific pattern to make human protein. Most meats and dairy products are complete-protein sources; eating fruits and vegetables in combination with grains makes these incomplete proteins more readily available to the body. Protein deficiency can result in lack of vigor and stamina, mental depression, weakness, poor resistance to infection, impaired wound healing and slow recovery from disease.

Carbohydrates   Carbohydrates are the chief source of energy for all body functions and muscular exertion and are necessary to assist in the digestion and assimilation of other foods. Carbohydrates fall into three main categories: sugars, starches (or complex carbohydrates), and cellulose.

Sugars, such as those in honey and table sugar, are simplest to digest and provide "quick energy." Complex carbohydrates found in cereals, pastas, and grains require more prolonged digestive action and provide the body with longer-lasting, more nutritionally-complete energy. Cellulose, the fibrous carbohydrate that makes up the skins of fruits and vegetables, is largely indigestible by humans, but provides the bulk needed for proper intestinal function and aids in elimination.

A total lack of carbohydrates in the diet produces loss of energy, depression, and breakdown of essential body proteins.

Fats   Literally the most fattening of food substances at 9 calories per gram, fats are essential to the storage of fat-soluble vitamins within the body and, through their insulating properties, to the maintenance of healthy, steady body temperature. Fat deposits surround, protect, and hold in place the organs— the kidneys, heart, and liver—and fat also rounds out the body's natural contours.

Saturated fats, found in animal meats and coconut oil, have been linked, when consumed at high levels, to an increased risk of heart disease. Unsaturated fats, derived from vegetables, nuts, or seeds such as corn, safflowers, and olives, seem to lower a man's risk of heart disease as well as keeping the skin and other tissues lubricated from the inside out. Adequate intake of linoleic acid, an essential fatty acid found in vegetable oils, keeps the skin healthy looking by preventing dryness and scaliness. A severe deficiency of fatty acids can produce eczema or other dry skin disorders.

VITAMINS:
WHO NEEDS THEM?

Contrary to popular belief, vitamins alone cannot provide your body with energy or instant health. Vitamins **are** essential for the conversion of food into useful energy by the body tissues, the maintenance of healthy body metabolism and the replenishment of body structures (bones, organs, and tissues). While vitamin deficiencies are certainly dangerous, doctors today are seeing increasing cases of patients who are suffering from vitamin overdoses, caused by taking too many vitamin pills in the mistaken belief that if some is good for you, a lot is even better. The average healthy man who eats a balanced diet really needs no more than a basic once-a-day multivitamin/ mineral supplement to provide all his daily nutritional "insurance."

What may create a need for additional supplementation are certain illnesses, heavy cigarette smoking, or debilitation caused by old age. Despite the fact that vitamin pills are sold without prescription, there is no way for the layperson to diagnose what he or she really needs. Merely popping pills because there are attractive-sounding claims on the package not only can be a total waste of money, but can actually mask the seriousness of a possible disease, or cause symptoms mimicking a disease state (vitamin A overdose, for example, causes internal tumor-like growths). A much wiser way to choose the vitamin supplements that are right for you is by consulting a physician and/or a nutritionist, who will take a complete dietary history and perform any needed medical exams before offering you advice.

All vitamins fall into two groups: water- or fat-soluble. Water-soluble vitamins are excreted in the urine and sweat through the course of each day if they are not utilized; fat-soluble vitamins are stored in the body's fat cells, where, if oversupplemented, they can build up to dangerous levels. The eight B vitamins and vitamin C are water-soluble; the huge amounts of these vitamins taken by many Americans who think they are improving their health, notes one well-known doctor, "simply gives us the most expensive perspiration and urine in the world!" The fat-soluble vitamins A, D, E, and K don't need to be replenished to any degree beyond the amounts normally found in a daily, well-balanced eating plan—and doing so can be dangerous to your health.

Minerals, while stored in the body, can be depleted by physical and emotional stress. The minerals present in the largest quantities (known as macro-minerals) are calcium, chlorine, magnesium, phosphorus, potassium, sodium, and sulfur. Trace minerals (aluminum, cadmium, copper, fluoride, iodine, and lead) are found in the body in tiny but crucial amounts. Until

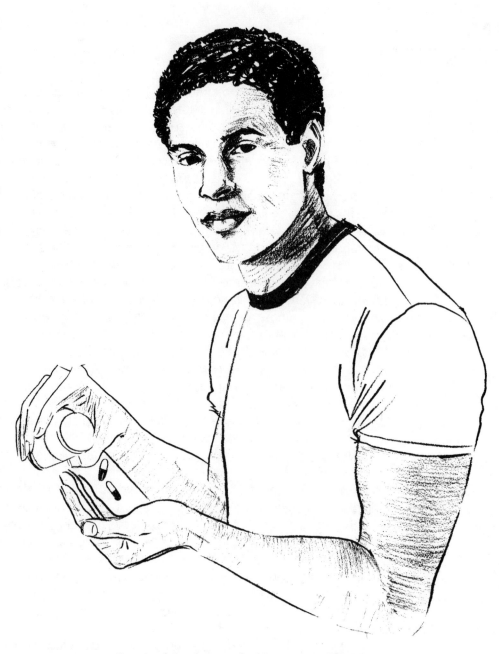

Beware of the dangers of taking too many vitamins.

recent years the function of trace minerals was not understood; today nutritionists have begun to understand their importance, as well as the danger of having too much of any particular mineral. Beware of unscrupulous promoters promising miraculous-sounding results from taking megadoses of vitamins or minerals; this practice can hurt your health more than it can help it.

Following is a quick summary of the role that the major vitamins and minerals play in the body, plus foods that are good sources of each:

Fat-soluble Vitamins   (Do not supplement unless under a medical doctor's advice.)

Vitamin A is important in the growth and repair of tissues. Adequate vitamin A intake helps keep the skin smooth and infection-free. A deficiency can show up as exceedingly rough, dry skin, ridging or peeling fingernails or even blackheads in some cases. Good sources for this vitamin are: eggs, cheese, yellow/orange/dark green vegetables, including carrots, broccoli, spinach, and liver. (Note: eating too many vitamin A-rich vegetables like carrots can give the skin a yellowish, jaundice-like tinge. Although not dangerous in itself, this can be a precursor or signal of vitamin A toxicity.)

Vitamin D aids in the formation and maintenance of healthy teeth and bones by helping the body in the absorption of calcium and phosphorus. Good sources are milk, egg yolks, liver, tuna, and salmon.

Vitamin E plays a role in the cells' ability to utilize oxygen as well as in healthy circulation. Deficiency is often manifested in dry, itchy skin or poor scar formation. It has never been proven that taking high doses of vitamin E will keep a man young, increase his virility, or do any of the other miracles often claimed! Vitamin E should, though, be a part of a healthy diet. Good sources are cold-pressed vegetable oils (especially wheat-germ oil and corn-oil margarine), raw seeds and nuts, green, leafy vegetables and whole-grain cereals.

Vitamin K is essential to overall health. Vitamin K deficiency is extremely rare as it is needed in such small amounts and is found in a wide variety of foods ranging from green, leafy vegetables to cabbage, cauliflower, and potatoes as well as cereals, yogurt, and egg yolks.

Water-soluble Vitamins   While these are not stored by the body and require daily replenishment, they are readily available within a balanced diet and do not need to be taken in high doses.

B-vitamins, which some experts feel are depleted by stress, help the body to process food energy and are thought to contribute to a healthy-looking complexion. Deficiencies can cause dry, red, cracking skin, especially around the edges of the nose and the lips. Good sources are Brewer's yeast, liver, whole grain cereals, pork, peanuts, and leafy green vegetables.

Vitamin C, while it does assist the body in the healing process, has never been scientifically proven to be the magical cure-all certain people have felt it to be. Whether or not you take vitamin C supplements seems to have less influence on whether you catch a cold or the flu than how many other people around you are carrying germs around! In fact, drinking a single glass of orange juice each morning actually provides a man with all the vitamin C he'll need that day. Other good sources are citrus fruits, tomatoes, strawberries, melons, potatoes, green peppers, and dark-green vegetables.

Minerals

Dietary deficiencies of minerals are relatively rare in adult men, although women are often lacking in calcium and/or iron.

Calcium is used by the body to construct and maintain bones and teeth as well as to preserve cell membranes in muscles and arteries. Deficiencies show up in bone loss and poor healing of fractured or broken bones. Good sources are milk and dairy products, sardines, dark green vegetables, nuts, and figs.

Phosphorus plays a role in cell growth and repair. Good sources are meat, fish, fowl, eggs, dried peas and beans as well as milk products.

Magnesium prevents tooth decay and some skin disorders. It is found in leafy green vegetables, almonds, cashews, soybeans, and whole-grain breads and cereals.

Potassium helps to regulate the body's water balance in conjunction with sodium. Sources include oranges, bananas, dried fruits, meat, and peanut butter.

Iron is important in the production of hemoglobin, the blood constituent that prevents anemia, fights fatigue, and helps to maintain strong skin and nails. Good sources are red meat, egg yolks, green leafy vegetables, dried fruits, molasses, whole-grain and enriched breads.

Copper is needed for the healthy balance and structure of blood cells, as well as for the maintenance of even pigmentation of the hair. Sources are oysters, nuts, beef, pork liver, dried beans, and corn-oil margarine.

Zinc helps the body to regulate a wide variety of metabolic processes. It is found in red meats, eggs, poultry, seafood, milk, and whole-grain cereals.

Iodine helps regulate the thyroid gland, in turn influencing total body metabolism. Primary sources are seafood, iodized salt, and sea salt.

Fluoride helps prevent tooth decay as well as bone infection and disease. Many Americans obtain fluoride in their drinking water. Other sources include seafood and tea.

HEALTH FOODS?

As more than one nutrition expert has noted, "There are no such things as good or bad foods, only good or bad diets." While the growing number of health food stores can be seen as proof that Americans have become more concerned with the food they eat, there is no reason that a man who wants to eat healthfully must shop in a health food store.

It is essential wherever you shop that you read labels, choosing foods that are lower in sodium (salt) and fat, higher in energy-rich complex carbohydrates, essential vitamins and minerals. When possible, opt for fresh vegetables rather than the processed variety (if you are in a time bind, remember that frozen vegetables are lower in salt and preservatives, higher in vital nutrients than most canned options). And be aware that smoked cheeses or meats contain more salt than other choices. Prepared salad dressings are higher in fat and salt than a homemade blend of mostly vinegar with a touch of oil, or lemon juice and vinegar.

As for sweets, don't be fooled into thinking that those made with natural honey are any better than those made with processed sugar. The number of calories may actually be higher without any more nutritional benefit in the long run! If you have a sweet tooth, try satisfying it with fresh strawberries, grapes, an orange or tangerine. That way, your body gets the benefit of added vitamins, minerals, and fiber as opposed to the "empty" calories of candy or cake.

WATER:
A SKIN AND HEALTH ESSENTIAL

If you've been searching for the secret potion that will help maintain health both internally and externally, and keep your skin supple, soft and youthful looking, you need look no further than your kitchen faucet. Water is nature's original beauty treatment—and our bodies need to replenish our interior reserves every day. In fact, you can survive a good deal longer without food than without water; the simplest thing you can do to improve your overall health and well-being, as well as the texture and tone of your skin, is to start drinking more water **now**.

A good daily guide is to consume eight or nine 8-ounce glasses a day. But all your water intake needn't be from a glass. Many foods have high water contents—apples are about 85 percent water, broccoli, celery, and lettuce each over 90 percent, green beans and aptly-named watermelon about 93 percent H_2O. Fruit juices are also good water sources; caffeine-containing beverages, however, tend to act as diuretics, robbing your body of fluids rather than supplementing them. A better substitute is caffeine-free herbal teas.

Why is water so important? To begin with, every cell of the body requires water in its essential structure and function. Water is the body's digestive solvent, moving food through the digestive tract and carrying fuel

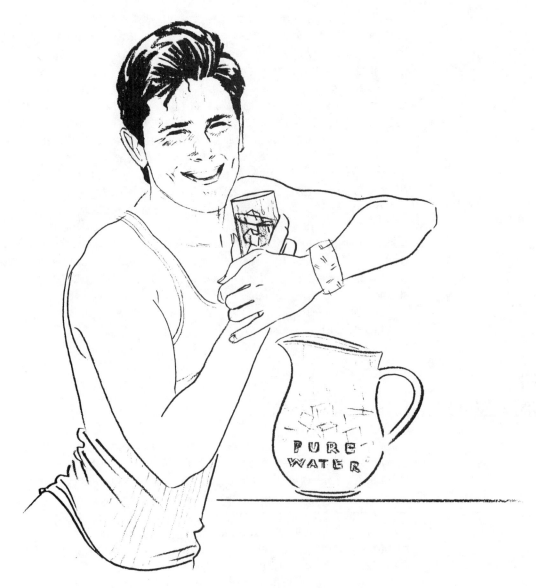

Water: It's the number-one health drink!

to the body cells, then carrying away wastes. In addition, water acts as a lubricant between cells, blood vessels, joints and internal organs. Our body temperature is maintained at a constant level thanks to our internal fluid balance and the processes of respiration and perspiration.

The skin is a major beneficiary of water's restorative powers, literally receiving moisturizing from within.The truth is that no matter how many different creams and lotions you apply from outside, they can only work by holding in the inner moisture your skin draws from inside the body, a fact too few men understand. Water is carried to the skin cells via the blood vessels much as it is transported through a pipe into your house. Water is the secret of both the texture and feel of the skin; without sufficient moisture the skin cells become flat, dull, and dehydrated. Water "pumped" from within plumps up the cells and gives the illusion of filling in tiny, dry surface lines.

WEIGHT LOSS:
WHAT IT MEANS TO YOUR SKIN

It is estimated that as many as 60 to 70 million Americans are victims of excess body fat—and just about every family's dinner conversation concludes with one member of the family promising to start on a diet "tomorrow." When your turn at tomorrow comes, be aware that there are differences between simply going on yet another diet and taking that excess weight off for good.

The first thing you need to know if you want to shed extra pounds is this: Most diets that work very fast end very fast too, with the unhappy dieter usually gaining back even more than he lost! The only way to become a slimmer man is to start living like one, by eating less and exercising more, with the result that you use up the calories you take in rather than storing them as extra padding.

A wise dieter will look for a balanced eating plan that includes no less than 1200 calories daily (more for a large-boned man) and a wide variety of foods. Beware of diets that center on a single food or require elaborate changes from your usual way of eating; you'll be less likely to stick with it. A safe, realistic expectation of weight loss is no more than 2 to 3 pounds per week. Any more and the diet is endangering your health.

Remember that the biggest problem with losing weight is keeping it off. The goal of your weight-loss plan should be a lifelong commitment to a new way of eating, plus an understanding of your personal eating habits. For this reason, many men find group-oriented weight-loss plans very helpful, especially those with classes in behavior modification. More and more corporations now offer executives the services of professional nutritionists and dietitians who can provide individualized advice on making realistic dietary changes.

Avoid crash diets. Not only do they put excess stress on the heart, the digestive system, and overall metabolism, but they can also literally increase the speed of aging of your skin. Men who make a habit of crash dieting (not uncommon since crash diets do nothing to change your everyday eating habits) tend to look much older than men who keep their weight basically the same or who diet slowly. Gaining and losing quickly can cause a loss of moisture in the tissues, and stretching makes the skin sag, bag, and wrinkle, especially when the skin is restretched repeatedly. In an effort to lose weight as fast as possible, many men choose diet plans with very little water or fat, both crucial to maintaining a healthy complexion. Once the weight is lost, the skin has lost the elasticity needed to bounce back onto its slimmer frame again. Here's the best dieting advice I can offer a man, from the standpoint of gaining a healthy heart and lungs, good circulation, and youthful-looking skin: Choose the body "size" best suited to nature's design for you early in adulthood and make a worthwhile commitment to maintaining it. Your overall appearance and healthy skin glow will be all the better for it!

CHAPTER EIGHT
STRESS

Don't look back. Something
may be gaining on you.

—Leroy (Satchel) Paige

Stress. Tension. Anxiety. They've become facts of modern life. Words we are all too familiar with—and that seem to never go away. Some of us let our stress "all hang out," while others hide our turmoils within ourselves. All of us, it appears, find a certain amount of stress simply unavoidable.

Among the stresses many men encounter every day are driving to and from the office in stop-and-go rush-hour traffic, dashing off to get to an important business meeting on time, running to meet a friend downtown for lunch, missing a phone call from an important business associate because you were stuck on line at the bank, and racing home early to be on time for your son's or daughter's first school play. While these are sometimes classed as "bad" stresses, there are so-called "good" stresses, too: the stress of getting a promotion at work, of getting married, of moving to a new and bigger home, or of seeing the business you founded undergo rapid expansion—all experiences filled with almost equal parts of joy and nervous enthusiasm. Even exercise—in the long run one of the best antistress release mechanisms—can increase your daily stress ratio if you're caught in a particularly competitive game of tennis or racquetball.

Why, in a book about skin care, have I devoted an entire chapter to stress? Because research has shown that stress takes a definite toll on a man's physical, mental, and emotional well-being—all factors that, over time, can influence the health and appearance of a man's skin. At its most basic level, stress triggers the release of "alarm" hormones within the body, hormones that increase the body's ability to withstand unexpected "attack." In the case of emotional stress, these hormones are often stimulated into excess supply, with the result that they cause new symptoms, ranging from stress-related headaches to muscle tension to digestive problems, along with skin reactions ranging from dry, itchy rashes to acne-like blemishes or breakouts (see Chapter 4). Some studies have indicated that, in cases of severe emotional stress, some men may even experience premature baldness (a condition known as alopecia areata; see Chapter 13).

As a general rule, stress will increase your susceptibility to skin problems that you've experienced at some time in the past. Yet even for a man who has been lucky enough to have had a perfect complexion for most of his life, it may also trigger the appearance of skin rashes or eruptions for the very first time. A man whom I had known for ten years, who always seemed happy and relaxed, suddenly developed severely dry skin and visited me in my salon. After first telling me that everything was "OK, just your basic ups and downs of life," he later disclosed that he was nearing completion of settling what he considered to be "a very amicable divorce. You know, we're just both reviewing the lists of what goes to who, and it's just a few days till we make it all final." Suddenly, I knew the reason for his dry skin went beyond what type of soap or creams he was using. I could help his skin to look as trouble-free as possible for the time being, but what he really needed was the passage of that "old healer"—time. The reason: no divorce, no matter how routine, is pleasant. And while this man may not have wanted to admit it to himself, the past year of his life had been filled with a great deal of stress—stress that was showing up, as it often does, in the look of his skin.

A GUIDE FOR MEASURING YOUR STRESS PROFILE

While experts note that none of us would want to live a totally stress-free existence, in which life would have **no** surprises, **no** excitement, **no** up-and-down rhythm at all, there are certain events that are like little "red flags" of stress. These are events that, unlike the momentary aggravation of a late commuter train, do not dissipate within an hour or so, but continue to wreak havoc over time. Many experts agree that if you've experienced several of the following events within the past six months or so, you have been under a substantial degree of pressure, and are more likely to experience a stress-related illness or accidental injury now or in the near future.

- Has your spouse or "significant other" died?
- Have you become divorced or separated from your partner?
- Has a close relative died?
- Have you been hospitalized?
- Have you separated from your spouse and subsequently reunited?
- Has your wife become pregnant? (Even if you've been aiming for this, it triggers definite stress.)

- Have you been fired from your job or laid-off?
- Are you having troubles in your sexual relationships?
- Has your financial situation changed radically—for better or worse?
- Have you changed jobs?
- Have you had an important job-related success?
- Have you been traveling a good deal and experiencing "jet lag" on a frequent basis?
- Have you moved to a new city or even to a new house in another area of town?

If you answered yes to several of these questions, don't despair. Stress does not have to mean it's all downhill from here. Being under stress does mean **learning to relax,** to unwind, to "de-fuse." While there is no magic cure for stress, there are many proven ways to cut down on its ill effects—and even learn, in some cases, to use stress to your own personal advantage.

RELAXATION:
IT BEGINS WITH ATTITUDE

How often have you heard someone—or even yourself—say, "I need to learn to relax."? Relaxation is, to a large extent, "all in the mind." What's needed is a realization that, when it comes to your physical and emotional well-being, what you don't do is as important as what you do—the time you spend relaxing is as important as time devoted to other activities. The more that researchers try to uncover the essentials of a healthy and long life, the more importance they give to the necessity of rest and relaxation. Also important:

- **Learn to say no.** One common cause of stress "overload" is taking on too much for the time and resources available. There is a limit to everyone's capacity; people around you, rather than being angry with you, will appreciate your honesty if you let them know when you simply cannot take on another commitment. Of course, this assumes you are scheduling your time wisely and not waiting to the last minute to let someone know you're unavailable. (If you find yourself repeatedly taking on too much and literally cannot say no, you may be hiding from a deeper problem and should consider some form of counseling.)
- **Try to balance work with play.** It's an old adage but a good one. Learn to schedule "time out," time spent with family, with friends, or in pursuing a hobby. This kind of scheduled relaxation is as vital to your health as is any other item on your personal agenda.

• **Learn the art of loafing.** Busy men often feel guilty if they spend time doing nothing. Yet none of us can continue for very long at "high speed," unless we want to end up burning ourselves out. We all need to spend time alone, to sit and stare into the fireplace, to go for a walk that has no real destination, or simply to play with your dog or walk on the beach. Learning to take a breather from the hustle and bustle of life may be the best favor you can do for yourself.

• **Get enough sleep.** While scientists still don't understand precisely why, they do know that no one can remain in top form or stay healthy for long without a certain amount of sleep every night. Feeling tired and rundown may be your body's sign that it needs more refueling time. Try going to sleep a little earlier, or making time for short naps between coming home from the office and going out at night. (You'd be surprised at how many famous men, including Thomas Edison, relied on daily catnaps.) Repeated bouts of sleeplessness should be brought to a physician's attention, as they may be signs of a more serious problem.

• **Make time for exercise.** Here are some of the pleasurable "side effects" of regular physical activity: you'll feel more relaxed, more energetic, and more capable of dealing with the many demands of life around you. What's more, many men who take up a regular exercise activity report that they have less trouble sleeping and feel more awake each morning than they did before. (For more on how much exercise you need, and on exercise's effects on the skin, see Chapter 11.)

THE SKIN CARE SALON PLUS

At first thought, the notion of visiting a skin care specialist for anti-stress treatments may seem strange, but think again. In the best skin care salons, every effort is made to create a quiet, soothing environment. The rooms are painted in soft, unobtrusive colors; everything is clean and well-polished, with a minimum of decoration. Your treatment takes place in a quiet, private room. The lighting is soft, the noise level kept to an absolute mimimum. There may be classical music piped into the room. You are seated on a comfortable reclining chair with your feet up and shoes off. Your skin is cleansed, then steamed; your facial includes a gentle massage of your face, your neck, and your shoulders. Once the creams or lotions have been applied, you'll be left in the room alone, to close your eyes, breathe deeply, even drift off into a few minutes of peaceful sleep. No demands are being made of you; you can talk or remain silent. What more could you want?

Then you won't be surprised to hear that many of my clients tell me that the reason they come to my salon is for a mini-vacation ... to spend an hour "off" with no phones ringing, no distractions, nobody to focus on but themselves ... to have someone pamper them and give them the freedom to relax. One man even told me that he likes coming for monthly facials "because it's less expensive than a therapist—and helps my skin as well as my psyche!"

For many men, who are so used to doing things for other people—working to make money for their companies, providing for their families, giving advice to their children and loved ones—a visit to a skin care salon can be somewhat uncomfortable at first. Suddenly, all the service is focused on you; you are asked to do nothing more than relax. But believe me, I cannot even begin to keep track of how many times my male clients have exclaimed, "If I'd ever realized how relaxing this would be, I'd have been coming for facials years ago." Once a man becomes accustomed to the emotional calm he gains in a skin care salon—as well as the real improvements he sees in the texture and appearance of his skin—he is hard pressed to give it up. In fact, men who once scoffed at the notion of skin care often become my most dedicated skin care clients! And they gain more benefits than many women because they become even more committed to the importance of daily at-home care along with regular salon treatments.

NEXT-BEST: A MINI-SALON AT HOME

What if you can't find the time to get to a skin care salon, or live in a small town where it entails a good deal of travel simply to find one? You can create a mini-version of the relaxing salon treatments at home. What you'll need first is a room with no distractions, with soft lighting. You might want to take the phone off the hook or have other family members cover for you for an hour or so. Perhaps you and your spouse or partner will decide to give each other the following treatments, beginning with 15 minutes each of de-tensing massage, using a light cream or lotion applied to the skin first to cut down on skin friction and allow the movements of the massage to have a smoother flow. Avoid heavy oils, as these tend to clog the pores; a water-based emulsion-type lotion is a better choice.

Your at-home skin refreshment begins with clean skin. Use a cleansing lotion to remove surface oiliness and dirt; follow with several minutes of warm water splashes.

Steaming your face must always be done extra-gently at home, where you lack the sophisticated temperature-controlled steam machines found in the best salons. Boil a small pan of water and add 1 tablespoon of chamomile tea. Remove the water from the heat. Apply a moisturizer to your face and neck to protect skin and prevent broken capillaries. Cover your head with a clean towel and form a tent over the pan to prevent steam from escaping. (**Note:** The steam should feel warm, **not** burning hot.) Wait five minutes, then follow the steam treatment with one of the following masks appropriate to your skin type …

For Dry Skin   Try an avocado mask: Peel an avocado; wash it in lemon water (lemon juice diluted in water) to prevent discoloration, then mash by hand. Smooth onto face and neck and leave on for 10 to 15 minutes, closing your eyes and relaxing. Remove with warm, not hot, water.

For Oily Skin   Use a yeast mask: Dissolve enough dried yeast in warm water to make a thick paste. Apply to face; leave on for 15 to 20 minutes. Remove with warm water.

For Combination Skin   Try this "Johnny Apple Sage" Mask: Purée an apple and mix with 3 tablespoons honey and one scant handful of freshly chopped sage. Apply to your face; leave on for 15 minutes. Rinse with warm water.

Your hands and feet can benefit from relaxing treatments, too. Break open several capsules of vitamin E and apply the oil to your feet and hands; cover each foot and hand with a plastic bag; put your feet up on the sofa and relax for 10 to 15 minutes; rinse with warm water.

Come-Alive Skin Lotion

To follow a mask and reawaken your skin: Blend ½ cup freshly squeezed lemon juice, ½ cup ice cubes, 1 tablespoon olive oil and ½ cup distilled water. Apply to skin with cotton balls; let dry. Follow with moisture lotion.

What if you've no time for all these preparations, have just come home from a stress-filled day at the office, and have barely enough time to change your clothes and run out the door? Take 10 minutes to relax, refresh, refuel, and try the following pre-party eye brightener: Wet cotton balls with cold milk; apply to eyes; lie down on the couch and relax for 10 minutes. Remove the compresses, splash your face with cool water, and then get dressed. Guaranteed: You'll feel as if you've taken more than 10 minutes off the pressures of the day, and will be ready to go out and have a good time!

You must remember throughout the reading of this book that there are relaxation-boosting benefits to all sorts of skin care treatments. It is up to you to remember that you are worth it. Your long-term health as well as the vitality of your appearance depend on your devoting time to relaxation as well as to hard work. And that "inner glow" that translates outward into healthy-looking, shining skin begins with relaxation.

CHAPTER NINE

EXERCISE AND SPORTS

Early to bed and early to rise makes a man, healthy, wealthy and wise.

—Benjamin Franklin

We have become a nation of movers and shakers, of joggers, runners, weightlifters, and aerobic dancers. According to the U.S. Department of Health and Human Services' Health: United States 1983 report, more than 35 percent of American adults now do some sort of regular exercise—and millions more men are joining the ranks of "weekend athletes" using their leisure time for something quite a bit more active than watching other men play sports on TV!

Research suggests that not only does exercise build strong, taut bodies, and improve a man's body tone and appearance, but it also helps prevent heart disease, fight obesity, high blood pressure and diabetes, and actually helps release built-up tension and anxiety.

Exercise increases overall health; it's as simple as that. It firms our muscles, flexes our joints, keeps us in shape. A man who's in shape is less likely to succumb to unexpected illness—and more likely to heal better and quicker if he does develop illness or injury later in life.

EXERCISE: ULTIMATE SKIN ENERGIZER?

Some of the positive side effects experts are also seeing in exercisers include increased blood flow and improved circulation, more efficient body "fueling," and healthier-looking, healthier-feeling skin. It may turn out that exercise is literally, inside **and** out, the body's best anti-aging tonic. Some doctors suggest that the increased metabolism that results from exercise—and that makes it possible for exercise to burn off fat and calories—may also speed up nourishment of the skin cells, enabling the skin to "renew" itself faster and to keep itself looking younger. For now, one thing remains certain:

A man who takes up a regular physical activity program, who starts feeling more vibrant and energetic, is also more likely to notice a newly-pinkish "glow" to his skin, a brighter tone and tautness to his complexion.

HOW MUCH EXERCISE IS ENOUGH?

Just what is meant by the phrase "a regular exercise program"? For a member of the New York Jets football team, the answer may be several hours of jogging, of push-ups and football scrimmages daily, but for most men (as well as women) the optimal exercise routine seems to be something between 15 to 60 minutes of aerobic activity three to five times a week (30 minutes three times weekly is often the most practical solution), supplemented by strength and flexibility training.

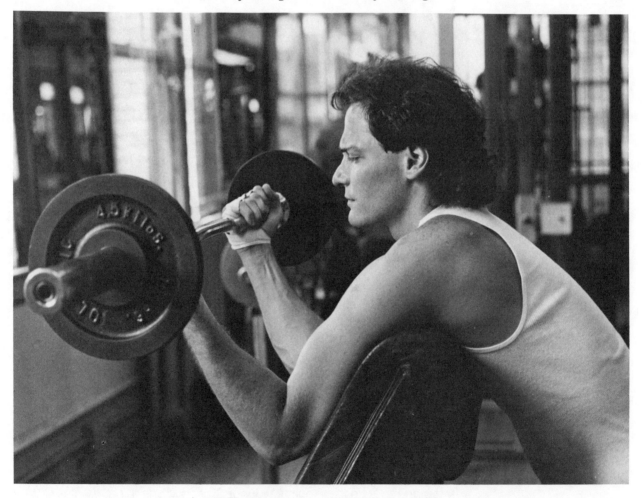

Pumping iron can change your skin-care profile.

What are the best aerobic activities to choose? According to the American College of Sports Medicine, aerobic exercise must work the heart and lungs, use the body's large muscle groups, and be an activity that can be maintained continuously and that is rhythmic in nature. Their top choices are: running, jogging, walking, hiking, swimming, skating (ice or roller), bicycling, rowing (in a boat or on a rowing machine), cross-country skiing, and jumping rope. Which activity you choose depends on a variety of factors, including which sport you most enjoy, what your current fitness level is, how old you are, how much you weigh, and the state of your overall health. You needn't do the same activity all the time; in fact, you may find it easier and more enjoyable to get exercise regularly if you alternate between different sports. One important consideration, though: if you are over 35 or have not done any exercise for several years, get a thorough physical checkup before beginning **any** exercise routine.

Other important components of total fitness are strength and flexibility. Weight lifting, with free weights or Nautilus or Universal machines, is a good choice for building muscle strength and endurance. Stretching (and warm-up and cool-down routines) will help increase muscle and joint flexibility as well as prevent injuries caused by pushing your body too hard when your muscles and joints are tight.

WORKING UP A SWEAT: THE GOOD AND BAD OF IT

Perspiration. It tells us our muscles are pumping, our bodies are working, the fat is burning. It is our skin's natural air-conditioning system, our bodies' natural self-cleansing mechanism. If left on the skin too long, perspiration can also turn into a powerful complexion-enemy.

Remember that the secret to making exercise work for your skin is to keep it protected from perspiration, not to keep it from perspiring. What this boils down to is this: cleansing your skin before **and** after exercise, using a moisturizer appropriate to your skin type, and keeping everything that comes into contact with your skin—your clothes, your hair, your sweatbands—as clean and bacteria-free as possible.

Perspiration is a mixture of water, body salts, and acidic waste products. While it is not true that only men sweat while women "glow," it is a fact that men's hormonal makeup increases the amount of perspiration they produce compared to a woman doing a similar level of physical activity. For this reason, men need to be even more conscientious when it comes to preventing sweat buildup on the skin's sensitive surface.

Although just about any soap will cleanse sweat off your body and underarm areas without causing much of a problem, the skin of a man's face is a good deal more delicate and requires a bit more care in cleansing. Whether your facial complexion is oily or dry, chances are you won't want to use the same detergent or deodorant soap you use on your body on your face.

SKIN FITNESS: CLEANSING PLUS PROTECTION

Here is a basic skin fitness routine for every exerciser, plus specific advice for the most common men's sports.

Before you start: Cleanse your face and neck, where skin is most sensitive, with a gentle cleansing lotion plus water; rinse well with splashes of warm-to-cool (not hot) water.

Don't shave right before exercise; its potential for irritating the skin multiplies when combined with perspiration. If you feel you absolutely must shave, use an electric (not a blade) razor and forget about after-shave lotion. You don't want the after-shave's alcohol content to combine with perspiration later. Instead, use a light, fragrance-free moisturizer to soothe and protect skin.

If you'll be exercising outdoors, apply a light moisturizer (this goes for oily as well as dry skin), preferably one with a built-in sunscreen. In cold weather (or windy conditions) a man with very dry skin will want to let the moisturizer set for five minutes, then reapply. In summer, always apply sunscreen lotion (the higher the SPF—sun protection factor—the safer your skin) wherever skin will be exposed.

If you'll be exercising indoors, in a gym with a high humidity factor, your skin will be thankful for it, even though you may feel a bit uncomfortable at first. The humidity will hold moisture in your skin and lessen perspiration's drying effects. Unless the air inside your gym—or your skin itself—is very dry, you should start your workout with freshly-cleaned skin and apply no moisturizing creams or oils.

Every exerciser should remember that where there's perspiration, there's evaporation. Since the greater part of our bodies are composed of and dependent on water, the water you lose during exercise needs replacing. Give your body a head start by drinking one or two glasses of water, fruit, or unsweetened vegetable juice before exercise, and take a water or juice break midway through your workout. Even the most highly trained marathon runners stop for liquid refreshment at water stations placed at roughly half-hour intervals; follow their example and you'll have a safer, more enjoyable workout.

During exercise, obviously you'll be focused more on pumping iron, scoring goals, or jumping higher than you will on the state of your skin. Still,

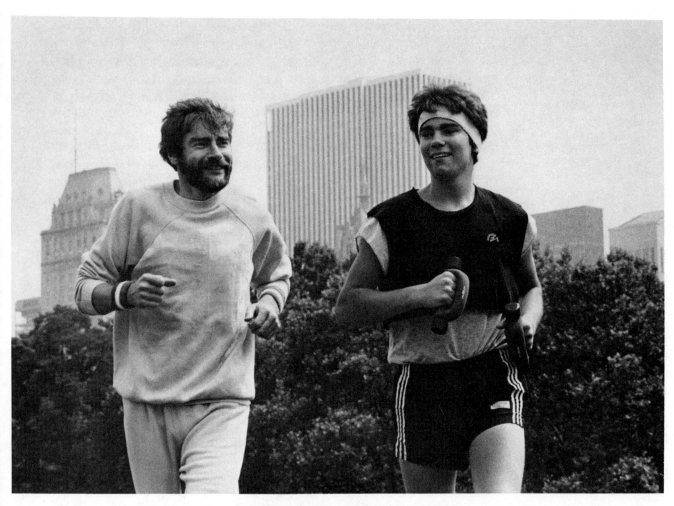

Outdoor exercise puts your skin to the test.

a few pointers can be helpful: If you perspire heavily, keep a towel handy to pat—not rub—some of the sweat away. If your skin is very oily, "arm" yourself with several cotton balls dipped in cleansing lotion to wash the perspiration from your face.

Post-Workout: Finish **every** exercise period with a cool-down, doing several minutes of stretching and gentle flexibility-boosting moves to calm pumped-up muscles and give your body a chance to rid your muscles of excess fluids and wastes. After your cool-down, head for the shower and turn up the warm (not too hot or cold) water. Don't overlook all-important cleansing spots like your shoulders and back, where perspiration can "pool" under clothing and cause breakouts later on. If you like the tingly-clean feel of using a cleansing sponge or loofah, now's the time to use one—but **never** on blemished or irritated areas, and **never** in a harsh rubbing motion. Don't use a loofah or harsh deodorant soap on your face; instead, use a cleansing lotion formulated for your skin type and rinse well, letting the water run down over your body and boost your after-exercise calm.

Finishing touches: Use a freshly-scented shampoo to cleanse your hair thoroughly, massaging your scalp in a soft, circular motion to cleanse away perspiration and dirt. (If you have a tendency to dandruff, choose a medicated shampoo, perhaps one of the newer formulas with built-in conditioning ingredients.) For last-minute invigoration, try a cool water head-to-toe rinse-off, then wrap your body in a big, fluffy towel and pat—don't rub—skin dry, dusting your skin with a fragrant talc afterward. As the final step, lavish a rich, creamy moisturizer on legs, arms, shoulders, and elbows, plus a lighter moisturizer on face and neck. Then it's time to reach for a tall, cool glass of water or fruit juice (or a mineral water/lime juice "cocktail" spiced with a sprig of mint) to replenish needed body fluids.

WHAT TO WEAR

Workout clothes are "hot." They are being worn not only to the health club or gym, but also to give a man an active image while shopping for groceries, heading for a casual date, or even simply walking the dog. Yet when it comes to maintaining skin health, the clothes you wear for exercise must fit their function as well as your body form. Here are some points to remember when you're choosing workout gear, whatever your sporting pleasure:

• **Wear loose-fitting natural-fiber clothing whenever possible.** Avoid tight-fitting clothes or fibers that don't "breathe"; these block perspiration from evaporating and cause uncomfortable and unsightly rashes. New high-tech fabrics are available that can actually keep an unexpected rain shower from penetrating your clothing but still allow perspiration to escape.

• **Keep your sweat clothes sweat-free.** Launder your workout gear regularly. The last thing you want to do is reintroduce bacteria onto the skin surface. This goes for headbands, wristbands, and chin-straps as well as T-shirts, sweat shirts, shorts, and jogging suits. If you're hiking or camping, watch for skin inflammation caused by an ill-fitting backpack or straps rubbing against sweat-moist skin.

• **Wear all-cotton socks.** Fungus infections such as athlete's foot thrive in dark, warm, moist environments—like inside sweaty socks. Cotton wicks away perspiration rather than concentrating it on skin surfaces as synthetics do. No matter how warm it is, always wear socks; damp sport shoes are optimum breeding grounds for infection. If the weather is particularly cold, layer several pairs of lightweight socks rather than wearing a single thick pair.

• **Replace your sport shoes before they're totally worn out.** All too often, athletes are so happy to have found the "perfect" shoes that they keep on wearing them long past their prime. Old shoes not only can cause blisters and foot soreness, but can throw your whole body off-balance as you move and cause eventual muscle or joint injury.

• **Watch for chafe points.** Don't buy activewear clothing that is too tight or has too much excess fabric at the skin's vulnerable points of contact—i.e., under the arms, between the legs, at the waistband. If irritation does occur, relieve the itchiness with cornstarch-and-water compresses (mix one-half cup cornstarch with one pint of cool-to-lukewarm water). Any rash that does not disappear within a few days, or that grows worse the second day rather than better, should be brought to a dermatologist's attention rather than self-treated.

SPORT SPECIFICS

Whatever game you play, following these simple guidelines will help improve the health and look of your skin, and make your sport more enjoyable and satisfying in the long run.

Swimming

• Chlorine and salt water both have a drying effect on the skin. Before taking the plunge outdoors, cover your skin from head to toe with a waterproof or water-resistant sunscreen (SPF 15 or higher is best; never use lower than SPF 10 when you're swimming). Don't forget the water-repellent lip-and-eye block, too. If you're swimming in an indoor pool, use a body moisturizer first to offset the drying effects.

• Your hair can suffer the same post-swim dryness as your skin. To get the best protection, apply a creamy conditioner before going into the water; follow up with post-shampoo conditioning later on.

• Take a shower immediately after swimming, even if it's just a clear-water total-body rinse-off. Take advantage of the pleasures of the outdoor showers found at many pools and beaches, but don't overlook the need to rinse your face and hair as well as your body. **Never** let irritating salt or chlorine dry on your skin.

• When you get inside, wash your face with a mild cleansing lotion. Splash repeatedly with lukewarm water, then apply moisturizer to face and body.

Jogging

• Always wear a sunscreen when jogging outdoors, as well as an eye-and-lip balm.

- Don't forget to protect **all** exposed skin areas—the tops of ears, back of the neck, shoulders, knees—from sun and wind with a high-SPF sunscreen.

- If your feet become sore or blistered, stop and rest. Check your shoes for signs of improper fit or excess wear.

Skiing

- Skiing combines the skin hazards of cold, windy, dry air with the sun-reflective danger of the snow. What's more, high-altitude conditions mean there is less air—and less pollution—to deflect some of the sun's damaging rays from your skin.

- Always be sure that your skin is thoroughly dry before heading outdoors. Damp skin is especially vulnerable to chapping and cracking.

- Use a high-SPF sunscreen whatever the weather. Clouds may block much of the sun's light but they don't block the invisible-but-burning ultraviolet rays.

- Wear dark-lensed, ultraviolet-blocking ski goggles to protect the eyes and the delicate skin around them from the sun. Preventing the need to squint will not only make your ski session more comfortable, but will also prevent the formation of the fine white lines at the outer eye corners and between the brows that are often the telltale marks of skier's sun damage.

- Wear a lip balm that is formulated with built-in emollients plus sunscreen.

- If your hands tend to chap and crack, apply a creamy moisturizer under your ski gloves.

- When you come indoors, avoid the skin "shock" of immediately sitting in front of a red-hot fireplace. Instead, take a few minutes to cleanse your face gently with a mild cleansing lotion and lukewarm water; if you take a shower, apply a heavy moisture cream to your face and body before **and** after. Once your skin is thoroughly lubricated, **then** go relax by the fire.

Tennis, Squash, Racquetball

- Always wear sunscreen when playing outdoors, applying a double-coating to nose and ears as well as to the often-overlooked backs of the hands (where sun-induced "age spots" often crop up first).

- If you wear sweatbands and wristbands, wash them after every game, just as you wash your face.

- Wear a sun visor to protect your eyes and the delicate skin around them from the glare of the sun.

• Between sets, pat perspiration off your skin with a clean towel and drink a glass of cool water.

Water-Skiing and Boating

• Be aware that sprays of salt water, plus sun reflection off the sand and the water, will be especially drying to the skin. Always apply water-repellent sun block to all exposed skin areas before you head outdoors; reapply every few hours.

• Pack a bag containing sun block, moisturizer, eye cream, lip balm, and—for cooling refreshment—a spritzer of cool mineral water to spray on the skin if you get too hot.

• Wear sunglasses and a hat while on the boat for extra sun protection; always reapply sunscreen when you come in from a water-skiing session.

• When you head for a post-boating shower, apply a heavy moisturizing lubricant cream **beforehand,** then reapply moisturizer when you step out of the shower as well, paying special attention to shoulders, elbows, and face.

Calisthenics, Aerobics, Weight Lifting

• Leave a window slightly open when exercising indoors to make it easier for sweat to evaporate off the skin surface.

• Never exercise with heavy creams or oils on the skin; a light moisturizing lotion is all even the driest complexion will need.

• If your exercise routine includes a good deal of jumping up and down, pay special attention to your feet after your post-workout shower: Pat dry, apply powder between the toes, plus extra moisturizing cream to the heels to reduce roughness.

Sauna and Steam Rooms

A few words of caution are necessary since sauna and steam rooms are often the last stop on a workout program.

• If you have sensitive skin, it's wise to avoid these rooms altogether, as heat can induce or exacerbate redness, worsen skin dehydration, and increase broken capillaries.

• To protect all skin types from heat-induced dehydration, keep your steam or sauna sessions short—say no more than five or ten minutes. Whatever your skin type, protect your eyelids and lips with protective moisture cream before entering a steam room or sauna.

• If your skin is dry, wash your face after exercising, apply a rich lubricant to face and neck, blotting off the excess and leaving on a thin film to provide skin protection. During the steam or sauna, massage additional moisturizer into your skin for "nourishment."

• If your skin is oily, cleanse your face after exercising, then use a grainy scrub (a cleanser with gentle abrasive ingredients), working it into the nose and chin, and leave it on during the sauna or steam session. When you come out, immediately rinse off the grainy scrub with lukewarm water, follow with a pore-tightening mask or cool-water splashes, and then apply a light moisturizing lotion.

A FINAL WORD: DON'T OVERDO IT

Just because regular exercise does wonders for the way you look and feel doesn't mean you should ignore signs that you may be doing too much exercise. Excessive muscle soreness or joint pain can be an omen of developing injury and should signal you to stop exercising and reduce your overall workout schedule. Any movement that causes sharp pain should be stopped. The professional athletes I see in my salon have learned this lesson well: Injury can be caused by carelessness or overdoing it at **every** fitness level, and a strained or sprained muscle can "sideline" even the most advanced sports players for weeks at a time. While these professional athletes often have the luxury of a masseuse and a physical therapist waiting in the locker room after each game, every sports enthusiast can create his own post- or pre-game relaxation. Here are my recipes for relaxation.

Post-Play Foot Soak

Fill a plastic tub with very warm water plus one cup of epsom salts. Soak feet for 15 minutes; pat dry with a clean, fluffy towel. Holding your toes, bend and rotate your ankle inward and outward several times; repeat with the other foot. Make a fist and, using a gentle circular motion, massage the sole of your foot; repeat with other foot. Starting at the toes, use both hands to slowly massage the entire foot, working back to the heel and up to the ankle; repeat, then do twice on other foot. Take each toe and gently pull upward and twist around gently. Apply a rich moisturizer, massaging it into the skin from ankles to your toes.

Hair Toner

To use as a final hair-and-scalp rinse after shampooing—Combine ½ cup white wine vinegar, ½ cup distilled water, and 2 tablespoons chamomile flowers (or loose chamomile tea). Boil for 15 minutes, then strain. Allow to cool; use as an after-shampoo refresher.

Skin Primer

The perfect post-exercise skin-refresher to have on hand in the refrigerator: Combine 1 tablespoon rosemary, 3 tablespoons chamomile flowers, 3 cups distilled water. Boil for 15 minutes. Strain; refrigerate. Use a cotton ball to pat on skin after perspiring.

Lavender Soak

The perfect post-sports bath—combine 2 tablespoons lavender flowers, 3 tablespoons bay leaves, 4 tablespoons fine oatmeal, and 4 tablespoons bran. Combine with water; simmer in covered pot for one hour. Strain; add to warm bath water; relax.

CHAPTER TEN

BAD
HABITS

Genius is one percent
inspiration and ninety-nine
percent perspiration.

—Thomas Alva Edison (1847–1931)

In a class I teach monthly on men's skin care, I routinely devote a section of the discussion to the habits that can have a deleterious effect on the skin: drinking too much alcohol, smoking cigarettes, abusing drugs, getting too little sleep because of partying late into the night. Without fail, at least one man in the group asks, "Does that mean that having good skin means I can't have fun anymore?"

I'm not here to lecture you on the necessity of a puritanical lifestyle. After all, what would having great looks, gorgeous skin, and a fit and trim physique be worth if you couldn't share them with anyone? The point I do want to make is that too much of the "high life" will not only eventually rob you of your health, but it will also rob you of your looks a great deal sooner. Overindulgence may be fun once in a while, but a man who wants to look his best and be mentally and physically at his prime needs to learn that "living clean is the best revenge." It's OK to cheat now and then, but pay attention to the need for moderation.

Let's take a closer look at the most common skin enemies and how to know when you're having too much.

ALCOHOL

Drinking is a very sensitive subject for many men; it can be harder to get a man in my salon to tell me about his drinking habits than just about any other aspect of his life. In some areas of business, the three-martini lunch is still very much alive—and the man who doesn't drink is more the exception than the rule. Pressure to conform, to have a drink with "the guys," can be subtle but all-pervasive. A young man concerned about his career prospects may feel awkward turning down a prelunch cocktail when everyone else, including his boss, is having one.

115

Yet this attitude is changing slowly but surely—and you can help to change it yourself. Perrier is now almost as widely available as Scotch, and even more chic in some quarters! As more and more men are watching their waistlines and becoming more conscious of maintaining their health, they are learning that cutting down on alcohol consumption is one of the simplest ways to cut down on calories. Consider these examples: An 8-ounce glass of beer contains 112 calories; a 3-ounce vodka martini 188 calories; a 1 ½-ounce shot of bourbon, Scotch, or gin about 105 calories. None of these contains any nutritional elements to help sustain your health! (Contrary to popular notions, the only "food" in beer is carbohydrates, the "simple sugars" rather than the more health-promoting "complex" kind, and wines—dry as well as sweet—are especially high in sugar.)

While it may be true that in your twenties you can "tie one on" at night and get up in the morning looking not all that much the worse for wear, once you hit your thirties your skin and your body begin to lose a good deal of their ability to bounce back from abuse that fast. You're likely to look—and feel—a mess.

How does alcohol affect your skin? For one thing, it acts as a vasoconstrictor, literally constricting the blood vessels and cutting back on the flow of oxygen and nourishment to the skin. This is the reason that an alcoholic is often distinguished by overconstricted, "broken" blood vessels on his face, although a person can drink a good deal less and develop a similar problem if his skin is highly sensitive. Second, alcohol is dehydrating, robbing the skin and other body organs of essential moisturization from within. Prolonged moisture loss eventually leads to fine lines and wrinkles, especially around the eyes. Excessive alcohol intake causes puffy eyes, blotchy skin, bloodshot eyes—not the notion of attractiveness to most men **or** women. Put simply, alcohol ages the skin and robs it of elasticity.

How much alcohol is too much? It's a very individual question. For a man with a fast metabolism, several sips can be all he needs to be making silly remarks or falling asleep at the table. For most men, more than one or two drinks a day is going to harm their appearance—and is a sign that they're probably drinking for more than mere relaxation. While some studies have shown that a man who has one drink a day is less likely to suffer from a heart attack than one who doesn't drink at all, every doctor will tell you that that is **no** reason to take up the drinking habit. When it comes down to it, there is really no such thing as drinking to your health!

Here are some easy ways to begin cutting down: Order a drink plus a club soda at the same time, and keep diluting it as you go along. Switch from hard drinks to white wine or, better yet, a white wine spritzer. Substitute tonic water, club soda, or mineral water for your lunch hour cocktail and see if you don't get more done in your office that afternoon than you would have if you'd had an alcoholic beverage instead. It may be a switch you'd like

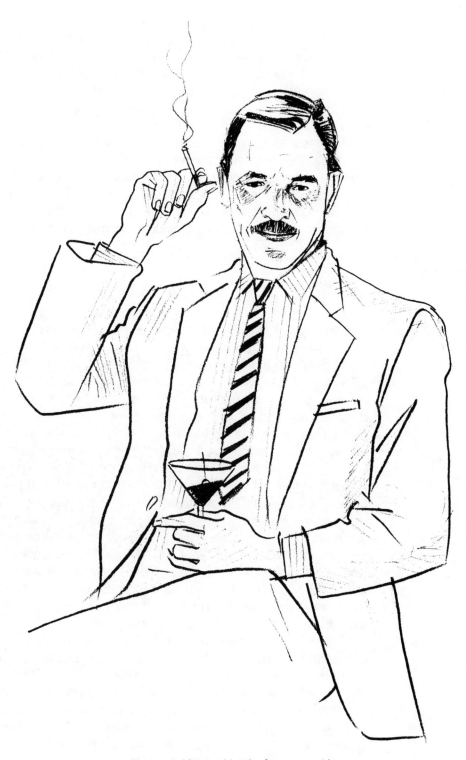

You can't hide bad habits from your skin.

to make permanently. Consider, too, new "nonalcoholic" beers like Moussy, which give you the taste—and the look—of beer without the after-effects.

If you know you're drinking too much but can't stop on your own, don't be shy about seeking help. There are many self-help groups, private doctors, and clinics that specialize in helping people cut down or stop their drinking habits. Realizing that you need help is the first, and often the hardest, part, but there is a lot of moral support around (see the appendix).

One note of caution: **Never** combine drinking with driving. More lives are lost each year in alcohol-related motor vehicle accidents than due to any other causes on the roads. If possible, always avoid being on the roads on "big" drinking nights—New Year's Eve, July 4th, St. Patrick's Day—to protect you and your loved ones from others who may not be as wise.

CIGARETTES

By now, we've all heard about the serious hazards of smoking—the increased risks not only of lung cancer, but all cancers as well as of heart disease—but I'd like to give you my own personal view. When I was a member of the Israeli army, as in most armies, roughly 99 percent of the soldiers smoked. I had never had the desire to smoke, and managed to resist the peer pressure ... until later in life, when I was having some personal problems and feeling a bit insecure. I came up with the idea that I looked much more sophisticated with a cigarette in my mouth. I felt able to socialize, to interact, to talk to people I had been intimidated by if I had the cigarette in my hand. I still didn't like the taste—in fact, I never even inhaled!—but I did like the confidence smoking gave me. Until, that is, I became romantically involved with a man who was a heavy smoker and realized how absolutely awful smoke smelled, how it got into your clothes and made them smell stale even when they had just come back from the dry cleaners, how your fingers, your hair all reeked of old smoke. Suddenly I just **had** to give up smoking, because I knew I smelled the same way. And that's the reason you should too—if you won't do it for your health, which is a much more important reason, but one that too few of us like to give much thought to until something goes wrong.

New research shows that while lung cancer may be the major hazard of smoking, it is not the only one. Smoking increases your risk of getting just about every disease, because it tends to compound the dangers of other risk factors, be they severe over- or underweight, high blood pressure or diabetes.

Smoking also literally makes your skin age faster. The reason: the carbon monoxide in cigarette smoke has a greater affinity for hemoglobin (the oxygen-carrying red pigment in the blood) than oxygen does, so it simply displaces it. The skin then has less oxygen available to it, and less ability to build up and repair tissue. Smoking makes skin look ashen and "tired." A lack of oxygen in the skin also eventually leads to dehydration, and gives the skin a greenish tinge that just about every skin care expert can recognize as the skin of a smoker. A new study published in the **Journal of Plastic and Reconstructive Surgery** not only confirms smoking's deleterious effects on the skin but adds another dimension to the problem: A smoker who undergoes plastic surgery is 12 times as likely to suffer healing problems as a nonsmoker. For men with oily skin, cigarette smoke can clog the pores, from the inside as well as the outside. A patient of mine, who had been a moderate smoker for years, came to me complaining of a tendency to develop blackheads around his eyes. I was able to clean the pores on a regular basis as part of a facial, but the problem kept recurring. One day he finally decided to stop smoking. As if by magic, his blackheads disappeared. Within a few months, when his willpower lessened and he took up the cigarette habit again, his skin problem returned as well.

Cigarette smoke not only disturbs your body's regular rhythms from the inside, but acts as an external pollutant also, adhering to the skin surface like any other type of dirt. You don't need to be a smoker to be confronted with this unpleasantness; we are bombarded daily by other people's smoke wherever we go. The solution: sit in designated no-smoking areas whenever possible, now showing up in many offices along with restaurants, trains, and airplanes. If smoke is annoying to you, don't hesitate to ask friends **or** strangers (politely, of course) to extinguish their cigarettes. After all, inhaling other people's smoke, say some scientists, is as dangerous to your health as it is to theirs!

DRUGS

When I first came to the United States 15 years ago, I was convinced that everyone in this country must be desperately ill. Everywhere I looked, I saw pills being advertised in magazines, on television, being taken by health food junkies, nervous mothers, women and men with headaches or the slightest sign of a sniffle. I had never seen pills taken so liberally back in Israel, and I just couldn't understand it.

Today the abuse of prescription and illegal drugs has reached mammoth proportions and penetrated all classes of society and age groups. It may seem glamorous in some circles to be taking the "in" drug of the moment, be it cocaine, marijuana, or Valium, but if you are a man who wants to look and feel his best, be energetic, enthusiastic, genuinely "alive," then you'll stay away from drugs, unless they are prescribed by a physician to treat or cure a specific ailment or disease. I am not against taking medication for a real medical need, but I am most certainly not in favor of looking to pills or drugs as a source of fun.

If you feel you have a problem with drugs—and one that is beyond your own ability to control—then most certainly seek help from a local physician, drug clinic, or self-help group (see appendix). There is nothing to be ashamed of in acknowledging your problem; it is only those who refuse to face reality that are to be pitied. If you're smart enough to care about your health, you'll be strong enough to lick a problem before it destroys you.

LACK OF SLEEP

Adequate sleep is the ultimate beauty bath of the skin. There is no cream, no moisturizer, no lotion that can match it. Adequate rest gives the body a chance to unwind, refuel, and replenish itself—and nowhere is this as obvious as in the look and feel of a man's skin.

Think of the difference in your appearance on days after a good night's sleep, and on those days in which you haven't slept much, or stayed out late, or tossed and turned worrying about a problem. Chances are, if you're like most of us, you look at least five to ten years younger simply by ensuring that you have gotten a good night's rest. Your eyes are less puffy, your skin is clearer and has more of a glow when you are adequately rested. Lack of sleep can make the skin look tired and ashen, and rob the skin of its natural pinkish color.

Most people need at least six hours of sleep a night and many need eight. Just as even the hardest, most productive workers need a vacation, your body needs its rest. Don't think that you can fool your body into getting by on less than you need for very long.

During times of added stress or tension—of an exciting new change or a nervous occasion—you may find that you have trouble falling or staying asleep. This is perfectly normal; no one can turn himself off and on like a lightswitch. Try doing some gentle relaxation exercises—yoga or ballet moves, warm-up stretches—to calm your body and mind. Never do vigorous aerobics before bedtime; it will only rev you up, not get you ready for relaxation.

If sleep problems are persistent, consider consulting a physician, as they can be a signal of a more serious problem. One interesting note: men who exercise regularly report less problems sleeping and more satisfying sleep than do those who are sedentary, probably because their bodies have a better balance between activity and rest.

CHAPTER ELEVEN

OUTSIDE HELP: BOOSTING YOUR NATURAL ATTRACTIONS

The style is the man himself.

—George Louis Leclerc De Buffon

M en today are concerned about their appearance for personal **and** professional reasons. Not only do they want to look their best for the inner satisfaction it provides, but for the benefits it brings from others: attracting friends and lovers, making it easier to interact with business associates and clients. Part of this growing awareness of self-image among men everywhere is the new knowledge of the small steps a man can take to better his appearance. Men who visit my salon, for example, ask questions not only about skin cleansing but about "faking" a tan with a bronzer or trimming too-thick or too-bushy brows. More and more men, experts report, are inquiring about the ultimate de-aging benefits of plastic surgery. Even if they're not ready to go "all the way" with enhancing their looks, it seems, men do want the information!

"I know I'm vain," said one 50-ish gentleman in my salon. "But I also know that I feel better when I look better. And in my business of sales, where deals are made on a one-to-one basis, appearance is very important. I don't think there's anything wrong with wanting to be well-groomed." A decade ago, such an admission would have been "unmanly."

BRONZERS:
SAFER THAN SUN

The secret behind many a year-round tan is the use of a bronzing gel to supplement a small dose of sun exposure. While once used solely by actors and models, bronzing gels are now being used by corporate executives, construction workers, lawyers, and engineers. Ten years from now, as more and more men **and** women realize the inherent dangers of sun worship, I predict that 50 percent of Americans, male and female, will get their tans from a tube of bronzing gel.

"But I can't wear makeup!" I can hear you exclaiming. A bronzer is **not** makeup; it is nowhere near as heavy or skin-covering as a women's foundation. It is sheer, translucent, light on the skin, and totally natural-looking—even to a woman close enough to be kissing your cheek! Many of my most conservative clients surprise me by suggesting that I tell them about bronzers, because they have noticed that a man at the gym or the office seems to look a lot tanner than they've ever remembered, and it turns out he is using a bronzing gel. The reason: in the two seconds it takes to apply a bronzer, your skin looks as if you have spent hours in the sun, with none of the unwanted side effects.

"But a bronzer looks so dark and my skin is so pale. It will be so obvious!" you say. Untrue. A bronzer looks dark when it is in the tube, but it is so translucent that once you spread it on your skin it lets your own natural coloring shine through. Bronzers are meant for every skin tone and, because they are sheer and nongreasy, are also suitable for any type of skin—dry, combination, or oily.

Bronzers come in stick or tube form. I prefer the tube form, because these are lighter gel formulas while the sticks are more similar to heavier cream makeups. Start with a small amount squeezed onto the palm of your hand and rub onto your face with your fingertips. Be sure to blend well; you don't want any streakiness. Blend the bronzer out to the "edges" of your skin, to the hairline and chin so there is no line of demarcation. As bronzers are stains, be sure to apply yours before you put on your shirt—and to wash your hands afterward. Don't apply a bronzer right after shaving; it may contain fragrance that could irritate newly-shaved skin. Apply a soothing after-shave balm first; give it a few minutes to soothe your skin.

Bronzers won't perspire off or streak during the day, but they should be washed off before exercise as you don't want anything that could possibly clog your pores to be on your face if you're perspiring heavily. Beware of overusing a bronzer; you want a hint of a tan, not a dark-brown wooden look. If you have trouble applying a bronzer at first, step into a skin care salon or up to a department store "men's bar" located in the cosmetics department for a quick lesson.

SPOT TREATMENT:
COVERING BLEMISHES NATURALLY

Since a bronzer is translucent, it is not going to cover blemishes or skin discoloration. What you need is a tinted drying lotion—a medicated treatment that helps blemishes heal themselves while keeping them under cover. These are available in several shades to match different skin colors.

Always apply a tinted drying lotion to clean, dry skin. If you apply moisturizer each morning, put that on first and wait a few minutes for it to "set." Beware of using too much drying lotion; you don't want glops of medication on your face.

Never rub anything harshly onto reddened or "angry" blemishes. This will only make them worse. Instead, wait for the infection to subside before using a cover-up lotion. Avoid stick-type "cover creams," as these can contain heavy oils that will only further clog pores and add to breakouts.

If you are using a prescription ointment to clear up blemishes, always apply this underneath a tinted lotion. You want to target the medication right where the problem is!

COPING WITH STAGE MAKEUP

For models and actors, stage makeup is a way of life. It is a necessity for their job, but it is an irony to their skin. The same makeup that boosts your attractiveness on the stage or in photographs can also cause havoc on your skin, resulting in irritation and skin breakouts later on. Here is some special advice for those men who must wear makeup in order to make a living, based on my years of experience as a skin care expert and the many Broadway and Hollywood actors and fashion models who have visited my salon:

• Stage makeup is harsher and heavier than the products sold in department and drug stores. To protect your skin, always apply a thin layer of moisturizer under your makeup as a skin barrier. If possible, ask the makeup artist to use water-based foundation as opposed to the oil-based theatrical products; this will be "kinder" to your skin under the hot stage lights, especially if you have an oily complexion.

• Do not shave immediately before applying stage makeup, as this may cause irritation. If you have an early-morning rehearsal or film shooting, try to shave the night before, right before bedtime, to give your skin time to recover.

• Always remove all your makeup before going to sleep or before exercising. Stage makeup can "suffocate" your skin, clog the pores, and cause acne-like breakouts. Use a specially-formulated makeup remover, not soap, which can fail to remove all the makeup totally and leave a film of oil behind. Follow the use of makeup remover with a liquid cleanser and then pat on a light moisturizer.

• The bright lights of a stage or film set, combined with the pressures of performing, understandably often result in increased perspiration. Beware of tiny sweat breakouts that often occur at the "edges" of skin, around the hairline and the jawline. Don't overlook these spots during cleansing. If makeup "spreads" to the hairline, wash your hair with a gentle shampoo.

• If you develop an allergic reaction to makeup, don't ignore it and hope it will go away. It won't. To try to "sleuth out" the product that is causing the problem, stop using all makeup for a while until the reaction disappears, then reintroduce them to your skin one at a time. When the reaction reappears, chances are it is caused by the last product you added to your regime. Stop using this last product. If the reaction happens to reoccur, consult a dermatologist who can perform a more precise patch test to isolate the product or ingredient that is causing the allergy.

• If you must wear makeup almost every day, then treat yourself to the deep-cleaning benefits of a professional facial at least a few times a year. Your skin will thank you for it; it will look cleaner, brighter, more refreshed—and you will be spared the breakouts that haunt many actors because they fail to completely deep-clean their complexions.

• At home, practice the art of facial "deep cleansing." At the heart of this process is a steaming of the skin, which should be done once or twice a week depending on how often you wear stage makeup and how oily your complexion is. If you wear makeup every day or have very oily skin, you'll want to steam twice a week; if you wear makeup occasionally and tend to have a very dry, sensitive complexion, steam once a week.

While steaming has been touted as a "pore opener," this is not really the case. Facial pores do not open and close like a closet door; pores do not have muscles so they couldn't possibly accomplish this movement. Pores are like pathways to the lower levels of the skin—steaming, because it is a superhydrating treatment, does seem to soften the skin and make it easier for dirt to be swept out of the pores during cleansing. Steaming is not a substitute for daily cleansing, but a supplement to it.

Follow these guidelines for safe at-home facial steaming (if your skin tends to be sensitive, steam for a shorter period of time the first time to be sure that you do not cause irritation):

1. Cleanse your face as usual, then apply a light moisturizer to protect delicate skin capillaries and form a shield over delicate skin areas as you steam.
2. Fill a large bowl with boiling water. Add lemon juice or a soothing herb (chamomile, for example) if you wish, for added soothing and a fresh scent.
3. Drape a soft, clean Turkish towel over your head and shoulders in a tent-like fashion directly over the bowl.

4. Keep your face at least ten inches from the water (getting too close can mean broken capillaries or acne encouragement).

5. Steam for five minutes, opening the "tent" and coming up for fresh air every minute or two; remember never to put your face closer than ten inches away from the bowl.

6. Blot your face dry, then cleanse with a liquid cleanser and apply a rich moisturizer, rubbing skin very gently in a light massage-like movement.

• Treat your skin to a skin-nourishing and cleansing mask every other week. It will remove any makeup residue and "rev up" a tired complexion, leaving your skin glowingly refreshed. (If you wish to give yourself a mask at the same time as steaming, do so after the steaming, before applying moisturizer.)

Rich Plum Mask for Oily Skin

Gently boil six plums (skin and all) until soft. Mash and add 1 teaspoon almond oil. Leave on for ten minutes. Splash off with warm, then cool, water. Pat skin dry. Follow with a light moisturizer on dry skin areas.

Masque Magenta (for Dry/Tired Skin)

Mince one medium-size raw beet (in a food processor if you have one) and add a few drops of heavy cream. Blend well in a food processor or blender; mix to a smooth paste. Apply to face; leave on for 20 minutes. Rinse off with cool water. Pat skin dry and apply moisturizer.

• **Post-performance refresher for all skin types:** When you've no time for a mask, but want something to freshen your skin thoroughly after a hard day's work, here is a zesty lotion to have on hand to apply to the skin after throughly cleansing off your makeup: Find the darkest-leaved lettuce possible and boil the leaves in enough water to cover. Let the mixture cool and then strain out the liquid, throwing away the leaves. Add in the juice of one cucumber (liquified in a food processor or blender). Refrigerate and use on those nights when your skin—and your spirits—need some extra "oomph." Apply with sterile cotton balls; follow with moisturizer suited to your skin type.

Irritated skin does not have to be a hazard of the acting or modeling professions. Proper skin cleansing, moisturizing, and professional facials can offset the harshness and heaviness of stage makeup and make it possible for a man to look as spendidly attractive off the stage as he does on. It doesn't have to take a lot of time; the suggestions above should be tailored to your individual skin type and time demands.

NEW GROOMING OPTIONS

Sometimes the most effective look-changers are the salon services that few men know about and none of them discuss! What often happens in a skin care salon is that a man may know what he would like to change about his looks but may not know that there is a way to do it. A sensitive—and sensible—skin care expert can often suggest new possibilities to a man who is receptive to new ideas. Here are two illustrative tales, both of them true-to-life stories.

Problem:
Almost-Invisible Lashes

A steady client of mine who is a Wall Street banker has the most beautiful shade of pale, pale blond hair and very light blue eyes—so light that they seem almost to melt into his face at times. I had had a thought that could help him but had been almost afraid to suggest it for months. One day, when he was having a facial and we were chatting in a friendly manner I blurted out, "You know, your eyes would look wonderful if you had a lash tint." "A what?" he asked. A lash tint, I explained, involves applying a natural-based, nontoxic dye to the eye-lashes to deepen their color to a soft brown and give the eyes more depth of color. He was horrified and proclaimed, "that sort of thing is not for me!"

That night he went home and discussed the "funny thing that had happened at the skin care salon" with his wife. She convinced him that it was a great idea, that it couldn't hurt him to try it, that after all I had been giving him facials for quite a long time and his skin looked better than ever. He cautioned me, "Just leave the dye on for a few minutes. I don't want my lashes to be black—and I don't want my clients to be able to tell that anything has changed!" I did just what he asked, left the dye on for two minutes, then washed it off and let him look in the mirror. His lashes were a warm, natural-looking brown and he loved the results. His eyes looked bigger, more attractive. And he's been coming back for regular lash tints every other month since. No one but he and his wife really notice the difference, which is just what he wanted!

Problem:
Grown-Together Brows

Some men's eyebrows literally meet in the middle. They grow in an almost straight line across the forehead and give the face an angry, stern expression even when a man is not angry at all. While women who have a similar problem have the option of tweezing their brows, men's growth is often too heavy to make this a practical solution.

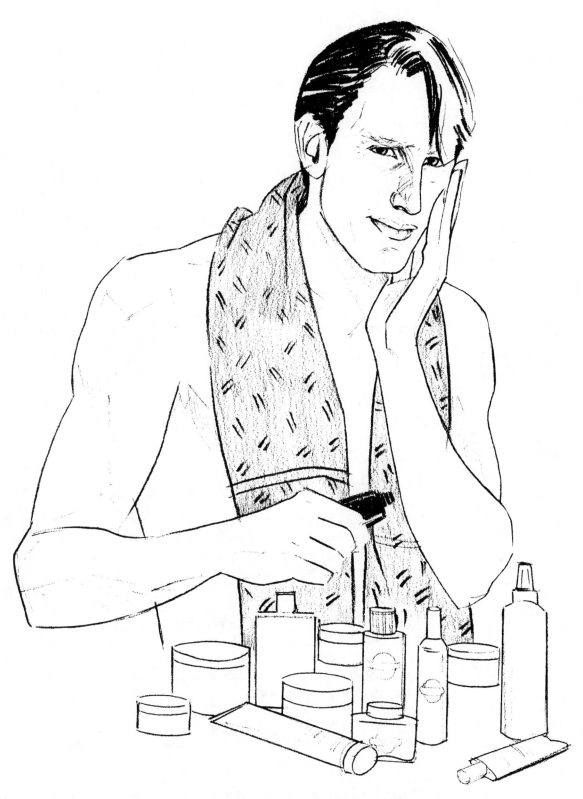

Skin care can be streamlined or complicated: It's up to you!

A "trick" some women have used for years and more and more men are trying is to wax the center of the brows by applying a warm, specially-formulated wax solution that whisks away the hair when dry.

When I suggested to one of my clients that he let me try waxing the midsection of his brows, his response was that it sounded like a good idea but he didn't want to become a slave to the skin care salon. I pointed out to him that the best thing about waxing is that it retards the regrowth of hair somewhat, and that he needn't commit himself to a regular schedule of waxing but simply come in whenever the regrowth got heavy enough that it bothered him. The best part of all is that waxing literally takes minutes.

The client let me try the waxing once, adored the results, and remarked that "my skin looks cleaner to me, my face more pleasing, and I have a new confidence in myself that must come from the inner feeling that I look better." Needless to say, he has been a steady waxing client ever since.

While these treatments are by no means for every man, they are just two examples of the options that a skin care expert can offer you, that you can discuss and consider without making an instant commitment to, and that illustrate the type of subtle changes in appearance that are the essence of attractiveness today.

ULTIMATE DE-AGING: PLASTIC SURGERY

What do you do if time has not been on your side, if you feel that you look so much older than you feel and would like to do something to turn back the clock a bit? One option that is appealing to more and more men is plastic surgery. Whereas once no man would admit to having surgery, today it is a topic that is being featured in more and more men's magazines, and is drawing inquiries from men all across the country, not just in the big urban centers of New York and Los Angeles. While I am not an advocate of plastic surgery for every man, I do feel that in properly-selected patients, surgery provides the extra edge in appearance that gives a man newfound confidence and acts as an inspiration to keep taking care of himself his whole life long.

Between 10 to 25 percent of all plastic surgery patients are now men, surgeons report. The reasons: "Job promotion, divorce, positive self-image, physical fitness; all these combined with today's accent on youth and health may motivate men. Many men view aesthetic, or cosmetic, surgery as professional insurance, helping them to resist competition from younger men, to gain a new position, promotion, or increase in annual income," reported Bernard L. Kaye, M.D., clinical professor of surgery (plastic) at the University of Florida and chief of plastic surgery at Baptist Medical Center in

Jacksonville, Florida at a seminar sponsored by the American Society of Plastic and Reconstructive Surgeons. "All things being equal, we unconsciously tend to pick the better looking person for the job. In today's professional milieu, the executive with a young face and body, coupled with the knowledge and experience time provides, is a first-rate contender with whom ambitious young men coming up in the ranks must compete."

Contrary to popular belief, most men seeking cosmetic surgery—like most women—are happy with themselves. They seek to improve their images, not to change them. In fact, some surgeons now report more and more "his-and-hers" surgery in which husbands and wives schedule simultaneous face lifts, have their surgery scheduled for the same day, share the same hospital room, help each other recuperate and, in effect, grow younger together. It is also not uncommon for one spouse's surgery to be so successful—and subtle—that it prompts the other spouse to schedule a consultation with a surgeon.

"In the last few years, it has become acceptable for men to admit to being concerned with their appearance. More than ever, men are concerned with looking and feeling good about themselves. This is evidenced by the selection of new styles and colors in clothes … the proliferation of hairstyling salons that have replaced the old barber shop," said Steven Herman, M.D., instructor of plastic surgery at Albert Einstein Medical College in New York City, who sees many male patients in his private practice. "Our youth-oriented society has made it increasingly desirable for men to look and feel younger. Cosmetic surgery for men has become an acceptable and popular means of obtaining a more youthful image."

A decade ago, the majority of men seeking aesthetic surgery asked for hair transplantation (more on this, see chapter 13). Today surgeons regularly see male patients requesting face lifts, eyelid surgery, nose reshaping (or "nose jobs"), and ear reduction. While at one time the only men who entered a plastic surgeon's office were actors, Hollywood celebrities, models or rich socialites, today the average plastic surgery patient is very much the average man—not overly rich or famous, but very much a "man on the street." Today men from all walks of life, especially the middle class, appear for consultations with plastic surgeons. Patients range from construction workers to athletes, military officers to lawyers, businessmen on all rungs of the corporate ladder. Some physicians report seeing increased numbers of schoolteachers among their patients, perhaps because men in such a profession are continually exposed to young people and are highly motivated to retain a vital and youthful appearance.

If you are considering plastic surgery, here are some questions to ask yourself before you make an appointment with a physician: Can you clearly define the change you would like to see made in your appearance? Are you realistic about the fact that surgery is surgery—that it has risks, limitations, and drawbacks? Are you happy with your present life or do you inwardly hope that having cosmetic surgery will instantly change your social life, your circle of friends, your business career? Is someone else pressuring you to have surgery? Are you under acute stress? If you are unsure about any of these answers, wait before seeing a surgeon. If you are hoping for surgery to be the "miracle cure" your life needs in terms of social and professional success, or if you are being pressured by a mother/wife/friend to have surgery that you don't really want, then don't bother going to see a surgeon. If you are experiencing emotional or psychological stress, then go to see a psychologist or psychiatrist before a plastic surgeon; you may still decide that you want plastic surgery in the end, but you should clear your mind of other problems first.

Before deciding that you want to have plastic surgery, you need to understand what specific procedures involve. Here are some brief descriptions of the most common plastic surgery procedures, based on conversations with Dr. Herman and other surgeons.

The Eyelift   "The earliest signs of aging on a man's face are often 'bags' or 'circles' around the eyes, which may appear as early as the thirties in a man who has an inherited tendency for such problems, or who has had repeated allergies that puff up the skin around the eyes, or has had a lot of sun damage in this area," noted Dr. Herman.

The eyes are the most expressive features, the feature most men notice first when they look in their mirrors, so it is not a surprise that eyes that look older than the rest of a man's face would be particularly disturbing. Having an eye lift won't make a man look twenty or thirty years younger, but it can help balance the eyes with the rest of the face, giving a man a more rested, refreshed look, adding a note of vitality to a man's face that may have been robbed over the years.

Usually both upper and lower lids are operated on at the same time, but they can also be done independently. The incision for the removal of "bags" above the eyes is made in the crease of the eyelid; the incision for the removal of excess skin under the eyes is made just below the lower lashes. Both incisions are designed to leave a minimum of scarring. If both upper and lower lids are done simultaneously, the operation takes from 60 to 90 minutes and is most commonly done nowadays in an in-office surgical facility (more on such facilities later). Patients return to the physician's office within three to four days after the surgery to have the stitches removed.

What will you look like right after the surgery? Bandages are usually applied right away but can be omitted if the patient has reservations about having his eyes covered. When the eyes are exposed, ice compresses (gauze pads or a cotton ball soaked in ice water) will need to be applied frequently during the first 36 hours. Your eyes will be puffy, swollen, black and blue—and generally look as if you've been punched in the eyes—for several days afterward. As with any surgery, you will have been given a local anesthetic and, in some cases, potent pain-killing medication from which it will take you about a day or so to recover. Many men return to business within a few days to a week after eyelid surgery, often wearing dark glasses for the first few days until the swelling and bruised look subsides.

The Face Lift   What a face lift can and can't do is often misunderstood. A face lift **can** remove sagging skin, excess folds of the cheeks and chin as well as folds of skin on the neck; it **cannot** correct fine lines and hatch marks caused by sun damage, which need to be treated by other means (see the section on collagen injections later in this chapter).

"Men are lucky when it comes to skin aging," says Dr. Herman. "Men usually don't need face lifts until about ten years later than women do because men's naturally thicker skin and shaving of facial hair prevents sagging to a certain degree. While the majority of women who come to discuss a face lift are in their fifties, we don't see men coming to a plastic surgeon to discuss a face lift until they are in their sixties in most cases. What is obvious today, though, is that men are taking better care of themselves. For many men, what prods them to want a face lift is that, because they are exercising more and eating less, their bodies are in great shape, and they just want their faces to look as healthy and full of vitality as their bodies do."

Face lifts are done somewhat differently in men and women; the primary difference is the placement of the incisions, considering men's differing hair growth patterns. No incision is made in the scalp above the ears because future hair loss could reveal such scars. There is also a naturally hairless area between the ear and the sideburn that must be preserved. Because men's hair is usually kept shorter than women's, the natural hairline is always maintained at the back of the neck.

The face lift incision begins at the front of the sideburn and goes back into the hair and across the back of the head parallel to the natural hairline. These changes in the incision do not make a man's face lift any less effective than a woman's, of course. Depending on the amount of sagging you have, this will alter the exact procedure.

Face lifts are done either in in-office surgical suites or in hospital facilities; this is a decision you can discuss with the surgeon you consult.

Don't expect to look wonderful immediately following the surgery. It will take a few weeks before the swelling and bruising disappear and your face looks as good as you expected. During the healing period, it is even possible for one side of your face to heal faster than the other and for the results to look "uneven." Don't panic; this is all part of your body's natural healing process.

Nose Jobs   For many young boys, an overly large nose is not only a source of personal embarrassment, but a subject of unkind teasing from other children. What we perceive as attractiveness is basically a balanced face—a nose that is too large seems to throw the whole face out of balance and make it unattractive. Often a too-big nose is simply a passing phase of childhood and as the boy's face matures, his nose seems to "fit" his face better. For others, a too-large nose never catches up with the face, and the young man may ask his parents if it is possible for him to have a "nose job." Where at one time the tendency was to do almost cookie-cutter lookalike nose jobs, nowadays surgeons stress that there is no such thing as a perfect nose—what is the ideal nose for each individual man is the nose that best fits his face.

Most of the growth of the nose has been achieved by age 15 or 16, and surgery may be performed from that age onward. Beyond middle age, you can still have nasal surgery, but the results will not be as good because your skin will not shrink back to your new nose size as much as it would at a younger age. The surgery may be done in an in-office surgical facility or in a hospital; local anesthesia is usually used and the physician will place a splint on your nose for about five days afterward. Packing will be put in the nose for the first few days, requiring breathing through the mouth.

"The type of nasal skin greatly affects the results of this type of surgery," says Dr. Herman. "Thin skin can be expected to shrink and thereby reveal the fine modeling of the nasal bones and cartilages after surgery. Thick skin simply cannot be expected to shrink in the same manner. This does not mean that a man with oily skin cannot have a nose job, but it does mean that he may not be able to achieve the same finely chiseled results as a man with thinner, dryer skin. In all cases, the desired result is a nose that appears natural and masculine and is in proportion to the other facial features. It should not be obvious that you had a nose job."

As all incisions are made inside the nose, there is usually no obvious scarring following surgery. In rare cases, where healing becomes a problem, you may have to return to the physician's office a few weeks later to correct small irregularities. There will be swelling and bruising around the eyes following surgery, and there may even be some swelling of the cheeks as well. Most of this disappears within a week, although there will be some subtle changes taking place for about six months to a year in the final contour of the nose.

Ear Surgery (Otoplasty)

While a girl can hide large ears under a long hairstyle, most men cannot. Young boys are frequently teased by their peers for having protruding or cauliflower ears. Approximately 90 percent of ear growth is reached by the age of five, so there is really no reason that a young child with unattractive ears must be made to suffer the emotional scars for the rest of his life.

Children are usually admitted to the hospital the day before such a procedure and go home the following morning. A light general anesthetic is used and a turban-type dressing is applied; this is worn for about a week afterward to make sleeping more comfortable and to protect the ears during the healing process. There may be some pain following the operation and pain medication is often made available by the physician. The incision is made on the back of the ear and cannot be noticed after surgery. The risks are minimal; bleeding and infection are extremely rare.

Adults are not "too old" to have protruding ears fixed and can often have the procedure done on an outpatient basis with local anesthesia. The face can be washed following surgery, although you will not be able to shower for about five days.

FINDING A PLASTIC SURGEON

One place to start is with your family physician, who can frequently give you the names of qualified surgeons in your area. Your local hospital, medical school, or medical society are also sources of referrals. A friend or family member who has had cosmetic surgery and is happy with the results is another possibility as is your local skin care expert, who may even be involved in follow-up skin care regimes for plastic surgery patients. The American Society of Plastic and Reconstructive Surgeons (write their Patient Referral Service, ASPRS, 233 North Michigan Avenue, Chicago, Illinois 60601) can provide you with names of board-certified plastic surgeons in your area who specialize in the procedure you are considering.

Questions to ask of any surgeon: Are you board-certified in the specialty of plastic surgery by the American Board of Plastic Surgery? Are you affiliated with a teaching hospital? (This is an indication that the surgeon has been recognized by his peers as worthy of teaching new plastic surgeons for the future.) How long have you been in practice? What procedures do you perform most often? (If you are having an eye lift, for example, you do not want to go to a plastic surgeon who rarely performs those procedures.)

Some surgeons will show you photographs of past patients during your initial consultation; others consider this somewhat unprofessional, as anyone who does show pictures will of course show you only his or her most successful cases. If you are shown photos, remember that each surgical procedure, like each person's face, is very individual, and that no surgeon, no matter how competent, can guarantee results. Not only is the surgeon's skill at work in the final results, but your body's own healing abilities are also at stake, something that is very hard to predict.

Seek out a surgeon who discusses the drawbacks and risks of any procedure with you along with its benefits. Beware of any doctor who repeatedly urges you to have more extensive surgery than you feel ready for. Be prepared to discuss possible side effects—bleeding, infection, swelling, pain—and feel free to ask any questions. Bear in mind that no surgery is without scars, but the aim of surgeons who practice cosmetic surgery is to make those scars as "invisible" as possible, so that they will not be readily visible to others. Plastic surgery is not as simple as changing your haircut or clothes; it is surgery, pure and simple.

Most surgeons require you have at least one consultation before actually committing yourself to scheduling your surgery. This consultation is **your** time to gain information and ask any questions you have, no matter how silly or simplistic they may seem. Some men feel that visiting more than one surgeon will help them decide who they want to trust with their surgery; others are so impressed by and confident in the first surgeon they consult that they go no further.

A note of caution: Recently several patients in my salon have asked me about getting so-called "preventative" face lifts. There is no such thing; getting a face lift before you need one means that you will not have very good or noticeable results. If there is no sagging skin to remove, there is no reason to "tighten" the face. The only way to prevent the need for a face lift in the future is to stay out of the sun as much as possible, and layer on sunscreens whenever you are outdoors. Genetics also play a very big role in how fast your skin will age, but this is an area over which few of us have much control!

Many men also ask how long plastic surgery will last, particularly eye lifts and face lifts. This is an almost impossible question to answer. On the one hand, cosmetic surgery will always put you ahead of the game and make you look younger than you would if you had never had the surgery. However, surgery does not stop the aging process, which starts up again as soon as the operation has been completed. Aging continues and varies from one person to another, but one thing is certain: Staying out of the sun will help any cosmetic surgery procedure to last longer than subjecting yourself to the aging effects of the sun.

SKIN SMOOTHING: MULTIPLE CHOICES

What bothers many men about their skin is not sagging skin but surface irregularities—fine lines above the mouth or around the eyes, depressed scars or differences in skin pigmentation. These types of skin problems do not disappear with a face lift but can be helped with one of the following procedures: a salon peel (see Chapter 14), dermabrasion, chemical peel, or collagen injections. The latter three can be done by either a dermatologist or a plastic surgeon.

Dermabrasion   This is a method of restoring wrinkled, scarred, or blemished skin to a more youthful, smooth appearance. A doctor uses fine wire brushes or a diamond abrasion sander literally to "plane" away the top layers of the skin, encouraging the growth of new, smoother skin to replace it.

This procedure can be either an out-patient (in the doctor's office) or hospital one. Depending on the extent of the treatment the skin may be left uncovered or a gauze dressing may be applied that, in a few days, will separate from the newly-forming skin on its own. Some doctors prescribe medicated ointment to be applied to the skin for the first few days. In any case, the skin will look raw, bloody, very much like a full-face friction burn or badly-scraped skin.

In a few days, the skin will appear taut and red, similar in many ways to a bad sunburn. As the newly-healed skin will eventually be slightly lighter than beforehand, sun protection becomes especially important once you have had a dermabrasion. You will burn more easily, tan less readily, and will need to use sunscreens with a higher SPF than beforehand. In fact, most doctors recommend that you stay out of the sun completely for the first six months following such a procedure.

Because it can result in loss of or uneven pigmentation, dermabrasion is usually not recommended for patients with black or olive complexions by many physicians, although there are some doctors who claim much success in using such procedures on darker complexions.

Chemical Peel Like a dermabrasion, a chemical peel aims at removing the top wrinkled or scarred layers of skin and replacing them with newly-healed, "younger" skin. In this case, a chemical solution is applied to the skin that literally "burns" away the top skin layers.

Some physicians apply a tape mask to the face after a chemical peel; others leave the skin exposed and prescribe an ointment to be applied. In any case, the skin will look raw and may be somewhat oozing for the first day or so. There may be some pain in the very beginning of the procedure, but the chemical solution itself quickly acts as an anesthetic, numbing the skin. Pain medication can be prescribed for those who are highly sensitive.

Extreme care in avoiding the sun is also necessary for some months following a chemical peel. As the skin heals after a dermabrasion or a chemical peel, some fine lines may reappear and the skin may not be perfectly smooth, but any lines will be much less severe than they were before the procedure was done. The skin may tingle or itch slightly during the healing process; pain relievers are often made available by the physician to use if needed. Some physicians recommend against chemical peels for black or olive-skinned men, as it may result in loss of pigmentation.

Collagen Injections Known as Zyderm collagen, collagen injections were approved by the FDA several years ago for use in "plumping up" depressed areas of skin, be they fine lines or the pitted scars that result from childhood acne. These injections can be used on fine forehead and smile lines, furrows between the brows, and depressed scarred areas.

Zyderm collagen is derived from bovine (cow) collagen that is processed to a highly purified state. Under the microscope, Zyderm collagen is almost exactly identical to the structure of human collagen, which is in part the reason that doctors have found the incidence of allergic reactions to the substance to be so rare. However, it is essential that every patient who is considering collagen injections have a test injection first (usually in the arm) to be sure that allergy does not occur.

Zyderm is packaged in sterilized needles and is injected into the skin by a dermatologist or plastic surgeon to fill in missing areas. Once it has been injected, it takes on the same consistency as body skin. Because it is packaged in a solution containing both saline solution and a local anesthetic, it is necessary for the physician to "overcorrect" the area at first, plumping up the skin more than necessary.

How long do collagen injections last? The answer ranges from six months in some patients to several years in others. Collagen does not stop the aging process; the lines may reform in the same area of the face that they did before but will probably be less severe than before the injections. Many patients return for follow-up booster injections within a year or two after their first collagen treatments. In the case of acne scarring, doctors have noted that Zyderm often seems to last longer, perhaps because scars are not as likely to reappear with the aging process as much as lines will.

One note here: Don't confuse the effects of collagen injections with that of moisturizing creams containing collagen. The collagen that is in a moisturizer stays on top of the skin to act as a barrier to moisture loss; its "plumping" effects, if any, will last several hours to a full day at most. Collagen in a cream cannot penetrate the skin in the same way that collagen injected into the skin by a physician can. Collagen is an excellent moisturizing ingredient though, because it has a natural affinity for water and helps to hold water in the skin and give it a smoother appearance. But there is no such thing as surgery in a jar; no such thing as an instant face lift. Be a smart skin care consumer and exercise common sense; it is the best skin care guide in the world.

CHAPTER TWELVE

BODY CARE: NEW SKIN FOCUS

By nature men are nearly alike; by practice, they get to be wide apart.

—Confucius

You run, jump, and pump iron to improve the look and tone of your body, but how much time do you devote to caring for the skin that is exposed to the hazards of perspiration, sun, and wind, in the gym, at the beach, and in some of life's most intimate moments? Chances are, if you're like most men, you think of skin care (if you think of it at all) as something that ends at the neckline. Yet men today, who take pride in staying fit, in maintaining physical as well as mental and emotional "strength," need to realize, too, that body care, far from being for women only, is an important part of being well-groomed.

Your body skin, like your facial skin, is constantly renewing itself. As new cells push their way up to the skin surface and prod old cells to slough off, dry, flaky patches often develop. In the back and chest areas, perspiration and oiliness can build up and cause acne breakouts, even in men who have otherwise clear complexions. Regular skin cleansing and replenishing moisturizing can help keep body skin in balance.

Just as small details often make the difference in the look of your clothes, small touches—the cleanliness and smooth shape of your fingernails, the "polish" of your body skin—are what differentiate a well-groomed man from the crowd. One of the nicest benefits of modern health-consciousness is that grooming rituals are increasingly streamlined, simplified, and hard-working. A man can take advantage of the chance to look his best without spending hours in front of the mirror. In other words, looking good doesn't mean you won't have time to do all the other activities that make up a modern, active life.

BACK FACTS: POSTURE PLUS...

It's the part of the anatomy every man depends on for support: ₊ne back. The irony is that, for most of us, it is also the body's weakest part. Attention to proper posture and carriage not only make sense from a health perspective; "walking tall" also helps a man to look more attractive, more confident, to carry his clothes better and to move with more ease and comfort. The muscles that support the spine include not only those of the back, however, but—perhaps even more importantly—those of the abdomen. Strengthening exercises aimed at the abdominal muscles, as well as flexibility moves aimed at the back, can help to protect these areas from injury and to maintain proper body alignment while sitting, standing, and moving.

The muscles of the back, especially those of the shoulders, are particularly vulnerable to tension. Nervousness, aggravation, and frustration all conspire to sneak the shoulders upward and tighten the muscles inward. Get into the habit of doing tension-relieving shoulder rolls at several points throughout your workday. Gently roll the shoulders forward and back...drop your head forward, stretching the neck muscles...breathe deeply...relax.

Posture and de-tensing work from the inside out; what helps from the outside in is careful cleansing and moisturizing.

The skin of the back tends to be the oiliest part of the body. Increased perspiration, plus a high concentration of hair follicles, mean that men are more prone to blemishes in this area than women. (Proof that every cloud has a silver lining: All this increased oil production means that your back will stay forever young—the skin will never wrinkle or sag!)

A hot bath can help dissolve oil and loosen skin impurities, but, ideally, it should be followed by a brisk shower to truly rinse off surface dirt and excess cleanser.

In the shower, apply a gentle foaming skin cleanser, using a back brush, natural bath sponge or washcloth (never rub blemished areas, though). Rinse well with warm, not burning hot, water. Then apply a gentle body scrub, softly massaging it into your skin using your fingers (or the fingers of a helpful friend) to buff away flaking skin and leave a finely polished skin surface.

Don't overlook the center of the back, where perspiration and bacteria can "pool" (a long-handled body brush can help to get at this area). Avoid using very harsh scrubs or loofahs on blemished skin, as this can spread infection. Do use a mud-based oil-absorbing cleanser, plus a medicated drying lotion, on these areas.

To keep back skin glowing, wear natural, cool cotton or other breathable fabrics next to your skin, especially when exercising. Follow cleansing with the application of a light, nonoily moisturizing lotion, always letting it set into the skin before putting on clothes. Launder your exercise clothes and towels frequently in a nonirritating detergent. In the sun, be certain to protect your back and shoulders (which often absorb much of the sun's heat and burning potential) using a high-SPF, oil-free sunscreen.

Treating yourself to a professional back "facial"—now offered at many of the best skin care salons—once every few months can be a wonderfully relaxing way to boost your back's appearance. It makes for a great transition from spring into summer, when you'll be showing off your body more. My male clients particularly appreciate the de-tensing benefits of the massage that forms a key part of every back treatment at my salon. Many tell me they are convinced that it even "relaxes" the skin of their faces, making them look younger all over!

YOUR BODY AND THE BATH

Through the ages, a bath has been more than just a way to get clean. Pliny reported the use of the bath as a medical treatment during five centuries in Rome; the Spartans of Greece expressed their "machismo" through a ritual of ice-cold bathing; and the Moors, who migrated to lush, green areas of Spain, expressed their appreciation for the magical pleasures of water by erecting luxurious, hauntingly beautiful bathing areas within the walls of the Palace of Alhambra.

While the number of women who take baths probably outnumbers those of men, more and more men are learning how relaxing an experience a bath can be—thanks, in large part, to the spread of hot tubs from the outdoors of California to the indoors environment of more and more houses and health clubs. Here are some pleasurable bath suggestions.

• For total relaxation, especially nice for a pre-bedtime bath, choose warm water (90 to 95° F), not hot. Hot water will only overdry your skin, and won't increase the skin-cleansing benefits. Warm water will, however, induce soothing circulation, help to de-tense tired muscles. For added skin softening, wrap some skin-smoothing bran, oatmeal, or almond meal in a cheesecloth pouch and drop it into the tub as it begins to fill up. If you want the addition of fragrance, tuck a few sprigs of rosemary into the pouch or add a few drops of essential oil to the bath water.

• For dry skin, warm baths are a better choice than hot; soft water better than hard. For a skin-smoothing milk bath (favored by Cleopatra, legend has it), add one or two cups of nonfat dry milk to the bath as the water is first filling up. Comfrey, marigold, or yarrow roots are soothing herbs that can be tied into a cheesecloth or muslin pouch and hung from the faucet as the water runs through. Extremely dry, flaky skin can get "ultimate" lubrication by slathering on baby or olive oil before you get into the bath, then soaking five minutes and gently rubbing your skin down with a loofah or body sponge.

• To soothe sore, tired muscles add a teaspoon of dry mustard or vinegar to the bath. Blackberry leaves, nettle, or eucalyptus tucked into a cheesecloth or muslin pouch infused into the bath like a teabag makes a muscle-relieving, body-stimulating tonic.

• Bath refreshers can turn a bath into reenergizing time-out. Turn the bath temperature down to tepid (80-85° F) and choose a stimulating herb infusion made from a mix of the following: basil, bay leaves, fennel, lemon verbena, or mint. Tie the dried herbs into a muslin or cheesecloth pouch and loop in under the faucet, letting the water run over the herbs as the tub fills up. Follow the bath with a cool shower. Be sure to consult your physician before taking hot baths if you are on medication, have high or low blood pressure, or have a heart condition.

• For every skin type, follow thorough back cleansing with a light application of moisturizer, letting it set on the skin before putting on your clothes.

STEAM AND SAUNA DELIGHTS

A steam bath or sauna can be the perfect post-exercise relaxer; followed by a cool shower, it can be an invigorating post-workout reenergizer. Be wary of claims of deep body-cleansing benefits of profuse sweating; what you lose through perspiration is primarily water, not body "toxins"—and your thirst will help you replace the water over time.

To make the most of a steam or sauna, keep this advice in mind:

• Check with your physician before "taking the heat."

• Always have a "buddy" take the steam or sauna with you to guard against falling asleep. It's best to stay in a steam room or sauna no longer than five minutes or so, especially if you're trying it out for the first time.

• Don't let the temperature rise over 115°F.

• A sauna is more drying to the skin than a steam bath. After either, take a shower and follow with a rich all-over body moisturizer.

• Boost the tranquility quotient of a sauna or steam bath by closing your eyes and slowing down your breathing (being sure, of course, that your "buddy" is close by).

YOUR HANDS: GROOMING EXPOSURE

Next to your face, your hands are the most exposed body part. And they definitely make an impression, every time you shake someone's hand, tap your fingers on the desk in impatience, or gesture to emphasize a point of conversation. Well-groomed hands are, in the end, what separates a "gentleman" above the crowd.

Today more and more men take advantage of the relaxation and grooming benefits of a professional manicure, now offered in many men's hair salons as well as in skin-care salons. Here is some advice for keeping your hands looking their best:

• **Use a hand moisturizer regularly.** This means in the morning before you leave the house and at bedtime, plus after washing your hands during the day, especially if you use a harsh commercial soap found in most office washrooms. Choose a hand cream that is not too watery but rubs into the skin easily (a lotion containing urea is a good choice), and keep a tube in your briefcase or desk drawer. Pay particular attention to moisturizing during cold winter months, and wear gloves to protect your hands outdoors. Rub a little extra cream into the cuticles and around the bases of your nails to keep them soft.

• **Clip nails straight across.** To avoid ingrown nails, clip nails in a straight line and use an emery board to file them to a subtly rounded shape. Use a soft nail brush to cleanse under nails daily.

• **To prevent dryness and cracking, use a gentle soap.** For use at home, a nondetergent bar or glycerine-based soap is the best choice; save harsh detergent bars for those days when you're greasing the auto! Liquid soaps are often a milder choice than bars; in winter, try to cut down on the number of washings and pay particular attention to moisturizing.

• **Wear protective work gloves.** Rubber gloves are good protection from harsh chemicals, dishwashing detergent (now as much a male hazard as a female one with so many men living alone or giving their wives some needed assistance!), and gardening dirt. To absorb perspiration and prevent skin irritation, look for gloves with cotton lining. If your skin is very dry, apply a rich waterproof ointment under the gloves.

• **Bring excessive dryness, redness, or cracking of the skin to a specialist's attention.** Sometimes rough, dry hands are caused by factors other than soap and the elements. Certain people, often those with a family history of allergy or asthma, may be predisposed to dry hands because their skin cannot hold moisture as well as it should. Redness can be a sign of dermititis, which can be further irritated by the use of moisturizers that contain fragrance additives. A doctor can prescribe a medicated ointment that will soothe the condition, rehydrate the skin and heal cracks or painful irritation. Afterward, once the skin has healed, be sure to use only hypo-allergenic, fragrance-free hand creams and lotions.

• **Treat yourself to an at-home hand smoothing massage.** Wash hands in warm water, then apply a gentle granulated skin scrub (the type you would use on your face) and massage it into your hands for a minute or two, beginning at the fingertips and working down toward the palms. Rinse with warm water, then apply a rich moisturizing cream.

FOOTCARE: BOTTOMS UP!

Whether you run, jog, play tennis or football—or don't do much more than walk to and from your car each day—you depend on your feet to take you where you're going. Yet few men pay much attention to their feet until they start to hurt. Treat your feet to a weekly soak followed by soothing massage and moisturizing. That way, you not only get a chance to relax and rest your feet a while, but you can also even prevent foot pain from ever occurring in the first place. Here is a quick at-home pedicure:

• Soak feet in warm, sudsy (use a favorite shampoo) water for five minutes.

• Use a pumice stone to gently smooth away rough spots.

• Apply cuticle remover to the base of the toenails.

• Gently push back cuticles with an orange stick.

• Rinse feet in clear cool water and dry carefully with a soft Turkish towel.

• Clip nails straight across; finish rough edges with an emery board.

• Smooth on a rich moisturizer, rubbing it into the skin with the pads of your fingers.

CHAPTER THIRTEEN

ALL ABOUT HAIR: FROM SCALP TO BEARDS TO MUSTACHES

What he hath scanted men in hair, he hath given them in wit.

—William Shakespeare,
The Comedy of Errors

A man's hair is literally his crowning glory. A healthy head of hair symbolizes strength, masculinity, and vitality. In literature as far back as **The Iliad,** mention is made of the beauty and thickness of man's hair, and it is little wonder the American Indians scalped their conquered foes to provide visual proof of their collective victories.

Changes in men's hairstyles have paralleled changes in the fabric of society as a whole. Our country's founding fathers wore powdered wigs to express their sagacity and position among the nobility or ruling classes. In the 1940s, men in and out of the armed forces sported crewcuts. In the 1950s, beatniks and rock stars like Elvis Presley shocked a more staid citizenry with their unkempt, less-shorn hairstyles, and in the 1960s, we saw the Beatles' cut everywhere—symptomatic of a whole nation's love affair with a four-man singing group. The hippie movement took the Beatles' cut a good several inches further, with men and women of the 1970s sporting ponytails and worried parents expressing the fear that it was getting impossible to tell the boys from the girls. In the 1980s, the dawning of a more conservative climate and the success of the "preppy look" have seen more and more young men returning to the close-cropped haircuts of their fathers' days, with a man whose hair touches his shoulders becoming a rare exception in most business circles.

The choice of a hairstyle is very personal, and it is not my aim to tell you how or when to cut your hair. One note of caution, though: Go to a professional to have your hair cut, as the true test of a style is not that it looks great when you leave the barber, but that it keeps looking great as you take care of your hair yourself. Where you go for a trim—an old-fashioned barber shop or a modern unisex salon complete with video fashion shows—is up to you, but be sure to choose a stylist who knows your hair's texture and the image you want to project, so that you get a style you feel comfortable with in the long run.

149

HAIR CARE: BEYOND BRUSHING

What makes your hair look good is not only the cut but how you care for it. The place that starts is with your choice of shampoo. In 1983, according to one consumer survey, men spent $142.6 million on hair products—and a good percentage of that went for shampoos.

Most men choose a shampoo because their mother or girlfriend uses it, they like the scent, the package, or the advertisement. In other words, for all the wrong reasons. Just as skin falls into different categories and has differing needs, so does hair. Depending on whether your hair is dry, normal or oily, look for a shampoo labeled accordingly. If you have a tendency to scalp flakes, try one of the new medicated shampoos that not only can correct but help prevent the problem (see the section on dandruff later in this chapter). Whatever type of hair you have, never use a bar of soap to clean it; it is too harsh and will lead to scalp dryness and flyaway hair.

How often do you need to shampoo? The answer depends on what type of hair you have and the kind of life you lead. A construction worker or carpenter who spends his days in an environment with dust and dirt flying around may find that he must wash his hair every day; an office worker may be able to get away with every-other-day shampooing. Exercise means perspiration—and perspiration means a need for immediate hairwashing. If your hair is very oily, daily shampooing will be a must. Men who move from the country to the city may find that they need to shampoo more often, once their hair comes into contact with increased pollution.

Every man, whatever his hair type or shampooing frequency, should use a conditioner to maintain his hair's shine and manageability. If you shampoo daily, it's probably a good idea to use an instant conditioner (one applied to hair, immediately rinsed out) after every shampoo. Treat your hair to an intensive conditioning every week or every other week, applying the conditioner, leaving it on for 15 to 20 minutes, then rinsing it out. Leave creme rinses for women; they are intended for long hair that gets tangled after shampooing.

Here are some more tips and truths on hair care:

• If you travel to different climates, you may need to switch shampoos. In greater humidity, for example, your hair may be frizzier, perhaps a bit oilier, and you may need to use a more conditioning but lighter shampoo. Many men also need to switch shampoos with the change of seasons, as they find that their hair gets dirtier-looking more quickly in summer compared to winter.

• Don't use heavy or greasy pommades on your hair. These products merely coat individual hair strands with oil. Instead, use a conditioner that penetrates the hair and fills in damaged or dry spots, lubricating and softening the hair over time. It is not uncommon for men who use greasy pommades to develop tiny acne-like breakouts around the hair line from these products, as they come into contact with the skin as well as the hair. If you feel that your hair needs styling help, try one of the new lighter conditioning gels or foam-in mousses, many of which contain built-in conditioning ingredients.

• Trimming your hair once a month or every six weeks not only keeps it looking neat but gives it a thicker look as well. Cutting off dry or split ends boosts hair's attractiveness, so don't neglect those haircuts!

• If you tend to perspire heavily, go for a style that directs your hair off the forehead to prevent perspiration from causing breakouts. Always brush hair off the face when washing your face in the morning and at night, and try to sleep with hair brushed off the forehead.

• Blowdrying may be part of helping your hair to keep its style, but it can cause hair to become dry and even break off at delicate points. Don't pull your hair tightly with a brush as you dry it; instead, hold the blowdryer six to seven inches away from hair and keep it moving from one part of the head to another as your hair dries. Use a diffuser when possible to decrease the intensity of heat and consider applying a conditioning spritz-type product to your hair before blowdrying.

• Avoid using a comb on your hair whenever possible. Combs rip at and tear hair and can irritate the scalp as well. Instead, use a natural bristle (boar) brush; plastic brush bristles often have rough edges that can tear delicate hair strands. "Comb" your hair into place using your fingers whenever possible, just use a brush to finish the styling. Also, be sure to shampoo your brush each time you do your hair to avoid spreading bacteria and dirt onto the hair and scalp.

• Rough towel drying is a no-no. It can break hair (hair that is wet is extra-vulnerable) and cause it to split or become damaged. Pat hair dry and let it air-dry whenever possible.

• Be aware that swimming in salt or chlorine water can be drying to hair as well as skin. Apply a conditioning gel or cream to the hair before going in for a swim and rinse hair with clear water right after swimming whenever possible. Watch out for the sun, too, which can bleach and dry your hair. Wear a hat or apply a conditioner containing a sunscreen whenever you'll be spending time outdoors.

• If you perm, straighten, or color your hair—as more and more men do today—be aware that all such chemical treatments can be damaging. Ask your stylist to give you a deep conditioning treatment first, and follow up with frequent at-home conditioning. Don't do such treatments too often, or your hair will look the worse for it.

● Many men now use hairspray. If you do, choose a product that is as light and nonsticky as possible and be sure that you shampoo out the spray that night. Beware of split ends or dry hair caused by hairspray buildup.

DANDRUFF: FIGHTING BACK

Most men assume that a dry, flaking scalp always indicates dandruff. Actually it can be the result of any of the following as well: an overall dry skin and scalp condition, shampoo residue left in the hair and not thoroughly rinsed out, or a sunburned scalp that is peeling.

If your scalp flaking is caused by a sunburn, you will simply have to wait until it heals. Meanwhile, frequent shampooing will help rinse the peeling skin away.

A dry scalp can be lubricated with a weekly olive or almond oil massage, which will also benefit dry hair as well. Apply olive or almond oil to the scalp with a saturated cotton ball. Put on a plastic shower cap to trap body heat and help the oil penetrate the scalp and hair. Leave the cap on for an hour or so or, if you are not a very restless sleeper, overnight. Shampoo the hair and scalp thoroughly afterward (two washings are probably best) and rinse repeatedly to remove all the oil.

Dandruff that does not respond to oil treatments may benefit from an astringent-type cleansing following shampooing. This is especially true if you have skin that tends to be oily, as dandruff may be the result of naturally-shedding skin cells that become glued together with excess sebum or oil. Mix equal parts of witch hazel and mouthwash and apply to the scalp with a cotton ball, following with a gentle massage. Shampoo and rinse well.

If these at-home treatments plus the use of an anti-dandruff shampoo don't solve the problem, then consult a skin care expert or a dermatologist, who can recommend more customized treatments. In cases in which dandruff is a recurrent condition, a dermatologist may prescribe a topical medication to be rubbed into the scalp following shampooing.

SCALP MASSAGE: SHOWER RELAXATION

To aid scalp cleansing and de-tense the muscles of the scalp, try this in-the-shower or -bath massage (for added pleasure, shower with a friend/your wife and give each other a scalp massage):

- Be sure nails are trimmed; hands are clean.

- Starting at the forehead, place both hands on your head, fingertips pressed to the forehead. Moving the fingers in small circular motions, work your way from the center of the forehead out to the temples. At the temples, lift your fingers and return to the center of the forehead. Repeat four or five times.

- Placing the fingers of one hand on your forehead and the fingers of the other on the back of your head, gently move your fingers back and forth, pushing the scalp gently in each direction. Repeat five times, changing hand positions so that the entire scalp gets the benefit of the massage.

- Place the hands on the sides of the scalp above the ears and massage as above. Repeat five times, using circular motions to the right and the left.

- Using the tips of the fingers of both hands, start at the base of the hairline in back (where your hair meets your neck) and gently massage the scalp in an upward direction, working your way up and over the top of the head to the front hairline. Repeat five or six times, slowing down the speed and decreasing the pressure of the massage each time to relax your muscles thoroughly.

- Rinse out shampoo and follow with an egg yolk conditioner (gently massage one egg yolk into the hair). Leave on for five to ten minutes and then rinse out. Rinse the egg out of your hair with lukewarm, then cool, water to leave hair shining and nourished.

GOING GRAY

Many men start spotting gray hairs in the mirror as early as in their twenties; it is not at all uncommon to see a man who has gone completely gray by his thirties. Not every man, though, is exactly thrilled to see gray hair in his mirror. A survey published in the February 1984 edition of **Product Marketing/ Cosmetics & Fragrance Retailing** magazine showed that men spent $28.9 million on at-home hair coloring products in 1983—a vast majority of that, I am sure, was for products that seek to cover gray. Millions more were spent in visits to salons for hair-coloring.

Does he, or doesn't he, you ask? One way to tell he does is if the color is not matched to his own, or if his hair takes on a flat, all-one-color look. Natural hair is composed of many subtly different tonalities—natural-looking haircolor must be too if you do not want it to look "fake." Consult a professional colorist (most consultations are free or available for a very nominal charge) to find out what coloring products will work best for you and produce the most natural-looking results. If you are using an at-home product, be sure to follow the instructions to the letter; most of the colorists will tell you that many of their most loyal salon clients first came to them to undo an at-home disaster!

Many of the most glamorous men are those who choose not to cover their gray hair, but to let nature take its course. As we get older, our skin color naturally gets a little paler, and lighter hair color (i.e., gray) can act as a "brightener." There is a certain air of wisdom, of life experience earned by a man who proudly sports gray hair, has a fit body and a confident spirit. Be aware, though, that gray hair can grow in more coarsely than your naturally darker hair, and you may need to switch your style somewhat. Proper conditioning and shampooing is, of course, still essential. A lemon juice rinse after shampooing can brighten dull hair and give it a shinier look.

Don't be afraid of gray hair and run to a bottle of color at the first sight of a few gray strands in the mirror. Give it a chance to grow in naturally before reaching for the hair dye; you may be pleasantly surprised at how distinguished and worldly you look. Chances are the women in your life will agree that gray hair makes you look not older but more handsome than ever. After all, Cary Grant didn't lose any of his sex appeal with his full head (and beard) of gray hair, so why should you?

LOSING IT:
COPING WITH BALDNESS

An estimated 20 million American men have some degree of baldness. About 40 percent of men between the ages of 18 and 29 are already beginning to lose some of their hair. Of the 60 percent of my clients who are men, about 10 to 15 percent are bald to some degree. In other words, if you are losing your hair, you are not alone. On behalf of myself and many other women, I would like to tell you that there is something incredibly sexy about a man of a "certain age" (yes, **your** age, whatever that is!) who may have lost much of his hair but is healthy, fit, energetic, in love with life and able to laugh, at jokes and even at himself.

There is no predicting at what age you may first begin losing your hair, but heredity has a lot to do with it. If both of your grandfathers, and your father and uncle, were all bald by age 50, chances are you may be too. Ronald Reagan obviously had a full-headed genetic background—in his seventies, the President of the United States still has a healthy mane of hair (although rumors abound as to whether its dark color is altogether natural). Others not so genetically gifted have made a career of being bare-headed— Telly Savalas and Yul Brenner among the acting set. Political success has come to many who did not sport a full head of hair—Winston Churchill, General and then President Eisenhower, Mayor Edward Koch, Moshe Dayan.

In short, losing your hair is nothing to panic about. Stress, many experts believe, can actually aggravate hair loss; worrying about your impending baldness may actually make the day come sooner when you no longer have your hair. Nutritional inadequacies can also be a contributing factor; a man needs a balanced diet for his body to carry out all its functions, including replenishing his head of hair (see the chapter on diet and nutrition). Rumors and miracle-claiming advertisements to the contrary, there is no vitamin pill or tonic that can restore a head of hair to the bald. Overall health, though, is essential. Extremely high fever, chemotherapy, and other drug treatments can cause temporary or permanent hair loss. Weather, while it is not a cause of hair loss or growth, does affect hair. Men and women lose more hair in summer than in winter, in hot weather than cold, as do all mammals. Shampooing doesn't increase hair falling; seeing a bunch of hairs collecting all at once in the drain simply dramatizes an obvious situation.

Scalp masques, given at many skin care salons, won't make hair grow but can give hair a thicker appearance, making it look as if you have more hair. They usually include a rich conditioning treatment plus a steaming, to help nourish the hair and the scalp.

COVERING UP:
STYLE OPTIONS…SHOULD YOU WEAR A TOUPEE?

While it is understandable and important that a man whose hair is thinning choose a hairstyle that makes the most of what hairs he does have, there seems to be some misunderstanding among some men as to how far such an effort should go. Too many men who suffer from thinning on the top of the head try to cover up this fact by growing extra-long hair on one side or at the back of the head and then brushing these strands up and over the top. Since these hairs are rarely thick or plentiful enough to truly cover the thinning area—and such efforts usually require strangely-placed off-center parts—the result looks very much like what it is: an effort at a cover-up. The man does not fool anyone and, in the event of a surprise gust of wind, can look quite foolish trying to replace his hair in the exact same configuration. Better than such contortions at the effort of covering the obvious: a consultation with a hair stylist, who can tell you the best way to style your hair, can give you a short, attractive cut that requires much less early-morning fussing and, while it may reveal a thinning or balding pate, does so in an appealing, natural-looking manner that can stand up to any weather!

What if you really dislike or feel uncomfortable about your progressive thinning? Should you try a toupee? If you have decided to, be aware that while a toupee may make you feel more comfortable, more youthful, or more presentable, no matter how high the quality of the toupee, it is usually obvious to others that it is not your real hair. If you do decide to wear a wig, don't try to cut corners by going for a less expensive version; when it comes to wigs, men **and** women get what they pay for, in terms of both quality and fit. Look for a toupee that is well-matched to your hair color and texture. If your natural hair is graying at the sides, then your toupee shouldn't be solid black, but should also be salt-and-pepper. Take your wig off in the evening; your scalp, like the rest of your skin, needs to "breathe" to be healthy and free of irritation.

It is usually a good idea to bring your toupee to your hairstylist so that he or she can show you how to "blend" it into your natural hairline and cut your remaining hair for the most natural-looking effect. Just as your skin color and haircolor change with age, you may not be able to wear the same toupee at 60 that you could at 40. If styles change, nothing will age you faster.

Follow the manufacturer's instructions for storing and cleaning the toupee. Wash it regularly, especially during the summer, when increased perspiration can cause a toupee to smell stale. Store the toupee as directed and replace it as soon as it stops looking fresh. If you find that it's uncomfortable to keep your toupee on when exercising, don't give up exercising; simply take the toupee off, spend the time concentrating on your fitness rather than your looks.

BEYOND WIGS:
HAIR TRANSPLANTS

An estimated 10,000 hair transplant operations are done by dermatologists and plastic surgeons each year, and the numbers are increasing. The reasons are not vanity or egomania but self-image, the desire of men who are balding to maintain their attractiveness and youthful look. While there are several different methods used by doctors, the basic procedures all have the same aim: to move hair from areas of the head where it is still healthy and growing (usually the sides and the back of the head) to scalp areas where it has "disappeared" (i.e., the front and the top of the head). The methods include "punch grafting" (in which plugs of hair are extracted from one area and inserted, surgically, in another), scalp reduction (in which the space between hair at the front and the back of the head is reduced), and hair transposition (in which strips of hair are moved from the back or sides of the hair to the front or top).

Whichever method the doctor recommends to you, be forewarned: hair transplantation is surgery, requiring local anesthesia in most cases (rarely, general anesthesia is used) and subject to the same risks and healing processes as other types of surgery. It is not always successful; some hair follicles may die in the transplantation process, a risk that is almost impossible for the doctor to prevent or predict. You may end up with less than gloriously thick hair after the transplantation—and it may take weeks or months for the transplant to reach its full growth potential, during which time your hair may look uneven or spotty in growth.

One important precaution: always have a qualified dermatological or plastic surgeon perform the transplant. Beware of artificial hair implants being advertised in many magazines and newspapers. In most cases, you will find that these implants are not inserted by a surgeon, but by a chiropractor or hairdresser. Doctors Vincent R. Digregorio and Gregory Rauscher reported in the October 1981 issue of the **Journal of Plastic and Reconstructive Surgery** that, while such implants often **seem** tremendously successful at first, they eventually result in infection, pain, loss of natural hair and degeneration of the surrounding scalp tissue in some cases. Such implants use not real hair but acrylic fibers meant for use in imitation furs and carpets, often stained with dyes that have been revealed to be cancer-causing agents. Surgery may be required to remove these implants and to restore infected scalp tissue. In short, the short-lived benefits of such artificial implants are far outweighed by the long-term risks of having such artificial fibers implanted in your scalp.

Hair weaving, another cosmetic alternative, is an option offered by some hairstylists. It involves weaving of synthetic or natural hair fibers into a man's remaining hair—and requires a good deal of remaining hair to be truly successful. When done properly on a man who is merely thinning rather than balding, it can produce satisfactory results, although the question of how long hair weaving will last depends on how often you wash or brush your hair. Hair weaving must be done very subtly and without producing undue pressure on existing hairs, and is a viable option only for those men who still have an equally-distributed amount of hair left.

Obviously, each alternative to balding has its pros and cons. A man might well consider the advantages of simply letting nature take its course. In dealing with men's vanity/sensitivity/emotions/life experiences every day, I know very well that there are many men who view the threat of balding as the worst thing that could happen to their self-images in the world. Some men can easily accept changes in their appearance over time; for others it becomes an emotional and psychological crisis. Remember, being a man is not only having hair; it is having a nice smile, a pleasing personality, a lot of caring and feeling inside. Being a man, too, entitles you to have a few scars, to have suffered a few bruises in your life and, eventually, to be bald. Attractiveness, more than any one feature or type of face, is a matter of attitude. And the sexiest man is not the one with the fullest head of hair, but with the nicest spirit inside!

FACE PROTECTION: BEARDS AND MUSTACHES

In ancient Egypt, as well as Turkey and India, a man's beard was regarded as a sign of dignity and wisdom. The longer the beard, the higher the man's rank and social stature. Mohammed urged his followers to grow beards, and to this day, the Sikhs of India are not permitted to remove a single hair from their bodies. Mustaches, too, have been symbols of adornment. The guardsman's mustache of the eighteenth and early nineteenth centuries was the sign of an army man, while after 1830 having a beard and mustache was a favorite affectation of the French radicals.

Some men still make social statements with their mustaches and beards (consider Salvador Dali-esque looks, for example), but most men use facial hair to achieve the same aims women do with cosmetics: to hide certain less-desirable features and emphasize the more attractive ones. Since a beard covers the bottom of the face, it focuses more attention on the top half, especially the eyes. A short, wide beard can add fullness to a long, thin face, while a jawline beard (à la Abraham Lincoln) can give strength to a weak chin. Beards can also downplay acne scars, make yellowish teeth look whiter by contrast, and balance the effect of a receding hairline. Beware of a beard if you are totally bald, or very round-faced; it will only emphasize both. Men who are especially sensitive to shaving or have a tendency to ingrown hairs might want to try growing a beard to give their faces a rest from shaving. But don't look at a beard or mustache as a vacation from grooming; to look neat, a beard or mustache must be trimmed and groomed regularly.

Beards and mustaches tend to go together, but it is possible to have one without the other. A mustache usually looks better on its own than does a beard; don't let one grow into the other, though, unless you're trying for a gorilla-like effect.

The biggest determining factor in growing a beard or mustache is your image. There is a certain mystery and devilishness to men with beards; facial hair must suit your total image and your character. Women are split on their reactions; some women love the look of a rough-hewn country boy with full beard and mustache, while others feel their skin getting irritated at the mere thought of kissing a man with a mustache. Don't grow a beard or mustache without at least warning your girlfriend or wife and getting some feedback; you may be surprised at her thoughts, and it's better to know sooner than later.

Different men not only look different with beards and mustaches; they literally grow and groom different versions. Think for a moment of Broadway and film heartthrob Jeremy Irons vs. supertenor Luciano Pavarotti vs. New York Mets Manager Davey Johnson, with his offbeat, longish mustache. You wouldn't mistake one of them for the other, in terms of personality, image, or career. A mustache and beard are as individual as their owners.

GROWING PAINS

The hardest part of growing a beard or a mustache, once you've made the decision to give it a try, is the first few weeks. Chances are you'll look pretty unpresentable, pretty scruffy for perhaps the first time in your adult life. (This is the reason so many beards are begun on vacation, when there's no one around to impress, no bosses to give you strange looks because you're seemingly unkempt.) Friends and work associates will be likely to tease you for your "attempt" to grow some facial hair. Other people may be worried that you're joining the Bowery gang. (One of my clients told me that he was frightening all the little old ladies in his apartment building when he first tried growing a beard—and you may be feeling as if you have!) New beards are itchy, to the grower as well as anyone close enough to whisper in your ear. They **feel** dirty because they cause you to keep scratching your face.

What you must remember at this stage is that patience is indeed a virtue. Don't shave at all for the first few weeks; you need to see the directions your hair grows in before doing any trimming or shaping of your mustache or beard. Keep the new growth as soft as possible with a cleansing lotion, rinsing with plenty of water and applying a moisturizer regularly.

Men with very curly hair may find that their problems with ingrown hairs persist during these first few weeks. Try to pull the end of the hair away from the skin **gently** with a tweezer; don't pluck out any hairs, though. If the problem persists, you might want to visit an electrologist for permanent removal of some of the most painful hairs (see Chapter 5 on shaving).

Don't begin trimming your beard until after about a month of growth has come in. But do keep shaving carefully—especially now that you have more time to concentrate on it—your neck area below the jawline. Once four weeks have passed, make an appointment with a good hair stylist who can give you a trained, objective view of the best beard and mustache shape for your face. Also rely on the stylist to do the first "shaping" of your beard and mustache, and follow his or her guidelines for future trimming. (Many of the neatest beards and mustaches are **always** trimmed by professional stylists, who have an eye for proportion and a steadier hand than most men.)

What if, even a month down the road, your beard looks patchy and uneven, with some spaces seemingly free of hair? You may be among the numerous men who can't grow a very good beard (there are more of these men than you may think) and who probably shouldn't grow one. The most attractive beards and mustaches are full and bushy, even if trimmed very short, and if yours just won't grow, there's nothing much you can do about it.

Some men shave their first efforts off and try again, in the hopes that their second growth will come in fuller. While this is sometimes true, in many cases it isn't. You may just find that the bearded or mustachioed look is not meant for you.

BEARD GROOMING

A beard, like the hair on your head, requires daily care. While the hair of a beard may hide blemishes or dry skin, it won't prevent these conditions—and the skin underneath still requires regular attention. Beard grooming involves not only the hair, but the skin under it.

To begin with, shampoo your beard daily, using a shampoo formula that is appropriate for your beard's hair type (in many cases, this may be different—drier or oilier—from the hair on your head). Cleanse the skin underneath your beard with a cleansing lotion (use cotton as in cleansing the rest of your face), then pat your skin dry with a soft towel and apply a light moisturizer to the skin. Gently brush your beard into the desired shape (usually brushing downward is best). Don't use alcohol-based colognes on your beard; they will dry out the hair and the skin underneath, and may even combine with perspiration to give your beard an unpleasant odor.

If the skin underneath your beard becomes dry and flaky, don't use a dandruff shampoo. Check to see that you are rinsing the shampoo and cleansing lotion thoroughly, and are using adequate moisture lotion. If flaking persists, see a skin care expert or dermatologist to diagnose the problem.

Your beard should be trimmed weekly. If you don't have it done professionally, do it carefully yourself using specially-designed beard scissors that you cleanse thoroughly after each use and store in a sterile place. Never cut your beard when it's wet; its curl or wave will make it look different, perhaps even lopsided, when it dries. Brush the beard up, then down, untangling snarls with your fingers, before you start snipping. Use a magnifying mirror; you want a nice, even line.

Always clean your beard after exercising. Perspiration can collect under the hairs and give your beard a "stale" odor.

If your beard comes in as a different color from the rest of your hair, you may want to trim it off. If there are just a few red hairs, say, sprinkled in a brown beard, then you can just snip these hairs out. Some men dye their beards, but this should always be done by a professional as it can cause skin irritations under the beard if not done properly. The exception: a salt-and-pepper beard, which can look very attractive on a man with mostly dark scalp hair. Of course, some men feel that gray hairs in their beards are aging, and may choose to shave theirs off if it comes in gray (for some reason, gray hairs may appear first in the beard rather than on the scalp).

MUSTACHE GROOMING

The secret of a well-groomed mustache is that no hairs should ever cover your top lip. After all, your mouth is a pathway in and out of the body for food and bacteria—and no one wants to kiss a mouth full of hair! It is especially unattractive when a man's mustache dips into his food as he eats, so never let your mustache get too long.

Always use clean mustache scissors to trim your mustache; don't let your mustache extend beyond the smile lines at each side of your mouth in width. Use a magnifying mirror to guide you to a straight line; if your hands are unsteady, have a barber trim your mustache.

Women or small children can get skin irritations from kissing a man with a mustache. If your spouse or kids express an uncomfortableness at kissing you once you've grown yours, you might want to consider shaving it off. After all, the ones you want to be most attractive to are the ones you love.

TAKING IT OFF

There comes a time when most men decide they're ready to try the bare-faced look again, be it for a new job or career change, or simply because they're ready for a new image or to return to their old one. You must be gentle when shaving a beard or mustache off. Not only is the hair of your face extremely strong, but the skin underneath will be extremely sensitive, as it has not been shaved in months or years.

Start by scissoring off the beard or mustache as close to the skin as you can. Then hop into the shower and douse your face with water before you even think about shaving. Apply a preshave softener, wait five to ten minutes, then apply a shaving cream (**not** an aerosol foam) and shave slowly and carefully. Use plenty of cream and a fresh blade. Don't shave the same spot twice. If your face needs a second going-over, start again with your preshave softener, cream, and a new blade (see Chapter 5 for the complete low-down on the proper shaving method). Follow your shave by patting (not rubbing) skin dry with a soft towel, applying an after-shave balm (**not** a high-alcohol cologne) and a rich moisturizer.

It's a good idea to shave off your mustache and beard on a Friday night, then let your face rest unshaven over the weekend till Monday morning. Your skin is likely to be quite tender and the beard area a bit paler than the rest of your skin. (Don't worry, this will soon go away and you won't be able to tell where your beard started or stopped.) Use the weekend as a skin vacation, allowing your skin to toughen up to the elements again without having to go through the hazard of shaving. Use plenty of moisturizer to soothe tender areas, and be sure to use a sunscreen with an SPF 15 if you're spending time outdoors, as the skin that was undercover for months will be very sun-sensitive.

Don't decide to shave off your beard on a whim, when you've had a little too much to drink or several nights without sleep. You'll just cut your skin to shreds and be sorry in the morning.

Do get a professional skin care consultation to analyze your skin type and be sure that you are using the proper cleansing products. It might be a good idea to go **before** you shave off your beard or mustache to get customized instructions on the right products to use and the best method to use to shave it off. Chances are your skin type may have changed between the time your beard was first starting out and when it's full-grown and off. You may need different skin care products now, and your skin could probably benefit from a deep-cleansing and nourishing facial. Let the skin care expert give you some face-saving tips. And bear in mind, while a 25-year-old's skin can easily recover from coming in and out from under a beard or mustache several times within a few years, once you've passed your thirties, your skin will more likely be a little slower in making a full comeback. Your main objective should be getting the right advice to make the most of your skin, whatever your age.

CHAPTER FOURTEEN

HANDSOME IS MORE THAN SKIN DEEP

> History is bright and fiction dull with homely men who have charmed women.
>
> —O. Henry (1862–1910)

Attractiveness is more than good looks. It is an attitude, a curiosity about life, and a desire for information. The kind of information that I have tried to provide throughout this book. Knowledge that can help you take care of yourself, enjoy life, and safeguard your health. This chapter gives you all you need to know to appreciate the benefits of getting a professional facial and convince you why it is something that every man deserves!

When I arrived in the United States 18 years ago, I was amazed at the lack of knowledge about skin care in this country among women **and** men. Americans were expert at buying products, being consumers of endless brands of soaps, deodorants, and moisturizers without knowing why they should buy one brand versus another. Men relied on their mothers, their wives, or their girlfriends to select most of their skin care supplies, as well as to decide what they needed to use. Rarely did a man use more than soap and shaving foam; hairspray was considered overdoing it as far as vanity was concerned. A man's idea of luxury was a horsehair shaving brush and soap-on-a-rope.

Today there's a shift in attitude, although there may still be some men who will hide this book in a brown paper wrapper. Major cosmetics companies are investing millions of dollars in developing and promoting skin care products especially for men. Fashion decisions for many men now involve much more than whether or not to wear pleats in their trousers, and some men are becoming as designer- and label-conscious as women are always accused of being. More and more men are trading in their glasses for contact lenses, not so much for improved vision as for appearance's sake.

In the late sixties and early seventies, when I worked in the men's section of a prestigious Madison Avenue skin care salon, the male clients were so intimidated by the idea of skin care that most of them—even the most loyal clients—came in through the back door. They always had excuses or explanations for being there, month after month. Their girlfriends had insisted on it, or their mothers had dragged them there, or they had received gift certificates for facials and just couldn't see them going to waste.

Today, men not only come to skin care salons across the country through the front door, but also have no reluctance in stating that they are there very much on their own, because they have decided that taking care of their skin is a worthwhile investment of time and money. Many of my first-time clients will tell me that they have read about me in a magazine, heard me speak on a radio show, or were referred to me by another man. They tell me that they have been wanting to take better care of their skin for a while, but have not known how, or where to go, to learn about skin care. They are curious about what an expert can tell them and eager to learn.

I'm not saying we've reached a time when every man proclaims his skin care allegiance proudly. Most men—and women—are a little nervous the first time they enter a skin care salon. They don't quite know what to expect. Some men dare me to prove to them that I know what I'm talking about; others are like shy little boys afraid to plunge into the pool off a diving board. Most of the time, they are very pleasantly surprised. They find that a skin care salon is not a place catering to mad egotists who think their appearances are the most important things in the world. I am not extolling vanity. What I am emphasizing, though, is a principle that every psychiatrist will confirm: The person who feels better about himself, who feels comfortable in his own body and with his looks, will be more at ease with himself and with others—and will be more likely to be successful in his business and personal dealings than will someone who is insecure about himself and his appearance. Going to a skin care expert is one way to boost your self-image and enhance your confidence and your well-being. I don't promise miracles, but I am here to help you.

SKIN CARE: IT'S LOGICAL!

Skin care is not magic; it is no more than a combination of knowledge of the biology of the skin combined with a large dose of common sense. If you're like most men, you wash your face at least twice a day, morning and night, and shave at least every other day, so why not take the time to find out the smartest methods and products to use?

In my 18 years of experience, I have given facials to movie stars, politicians, lawyers, accountants, construction workers, carpenters, truck drivers, and schoolteachers as well as writers, photographers, computer programmers, and salesmen. Regardless of their social backgrounds or incomes, whether they were happily married, single, or divorced, they all shared a desire to look their best and a need for a few minutes of relaxation every few weeks out of their busy lives. I have had businessmen in my salon who make million-dollar decisions every day of their lives, the type of men whom you would imagine would dismiss a facial as something for "sissies." Yet the more pressure a man has to put up with every day, the less time he thinks he has for himself, the more he needs the benefit of some time to himself, away from the ringing of telephones, the orders of your foreman or boss, the responsibility of running an office, a business, or a home.

A skin care specialist offers not only expertise but also the rare luxury of time for yourself, in which **you** are the focus of attention. While your skin is being cleansed and refreshed, you have had the time to clear your mind of the cares of the day, to start anew. Your visit to a skin care salon can be, in essence, a mini-vacation. There are some skin care problems a skin specialist should never treat, such as moles, severe acne, skin diseases and rashes. These should be brought to a dermatologist's attention.

LIA'S FACIAL: BEYOND PAMPERING

The essence of a top-notch facial is relaxed caring. The treatment must be customized to your skin's particular needs. A proper facial takes about an hour, a little shorter if your skin is problem-free, a little longer if your skin is very clogged or has been neglected. Some salons offer what they call "mini-facials," promising to have you in and out in under a half hour. I do not believe in these because you cannot possibly provide the thorough skin cleansing or relaxation that a true facial should include in that short time period. The more a skin care salon rushes the treatment, the greater the chances of your skin being irritated or mistreated in the process.

Step One: Skin Analysis
No facial should begin without a skin examination, first with the "naked eye," then under a magnifying lamp. The analysis will take a little longer on your first visit but should always be repeated on subsequent visits as your skin is alive and changing and could have undergone some changes between facials, for better or worse. The aim of subsequent analysis should also be for your skin care adviser to check whether your at-home skin care routine is working, and if it is helping to keep your skin in good "shape."

Step Two: Massage
As I said earlier, I believe that every facial should be relaxing, so the second step of every treatment in my salon is a de-tensing massage. Depending on your skin type, this step may combine a neck and shoulder massage with a gentle facial massage. If your skin is acne-prone or very dry and delicate, the massage would probably be limited to the neck and shoulders. The relaxing effects are not limited, though, to the areas being massaged. De-stressing

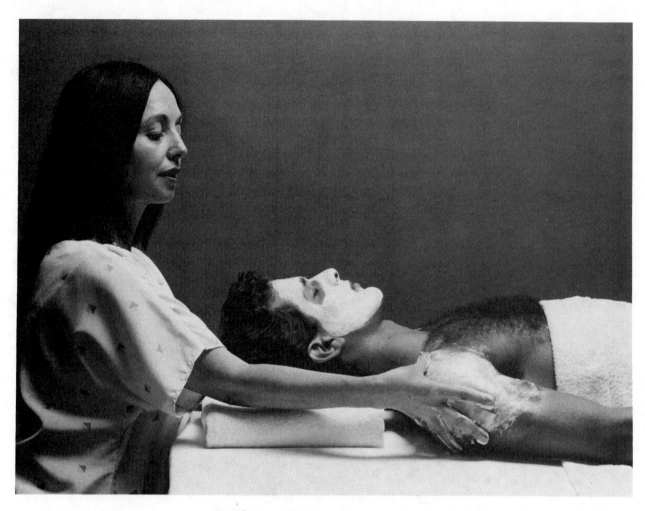

A professional facial: the ultimate skin luxury.

one area of the body has a wonderful carryover effect to the rest of the body, spreading the relaxation benefits. A 10- to 15-minute massage increases the circulation, relaxes the muscles, and prepares your skin to take advantage of the skin care benefits to come. Contrary to myth, massage does not break down or harm the skin if done correctly. Our facial muscles are constantly at work, moving our face into different expressions, helping us smile, frown, and talk; gentle massage gives them a rest and increases your comfort in the salon and afterward. In fact, many of my clients tell me that, to their minds, the massage is the best part of their facial!

Step Three: Skin-Steaming   Using an aromatic mixture of herbs and soothing plant essences selected especially for your skin type, then blended in a warm spring water steam infusion, I will steam the skin for about five minutes. This will soften and soothe the skin. Steaming should never be burning hot nor should it be done on bare, unprotected skin. A light moisturizer should always be applied first to protect the skin, and cool compresses should be placed over the eyes to soothe and protect them. A vaporizing type of steam machine is usually used. It's also important that a rich cream be smoothed over the neck to be left on throughout the facial.

Step Four: Cleansing

Once the skin has been softened, the skin care expert will cleanse the pores of oil and dirt, paying special attention to blackheads and whiteheads. An eye cream will be applied around the eyes, where no cleaning will be done unless absolutely necessary.

The cleansing should always be gentle. It should not be painful, although it may be a little uncomfortable if the pores are very clogged or you have been ill or had a fever or never had a facial before. Always ask the esthetician to stop immediately if something hurts you; he or she may not be aware of how sensitive your skin is (although a knowledgable expert should recognize this). Remember, the facial is for you; anything that feels uncomfortable should be brought to the salon's attention.

Step Five: Antiseptic

The cleansing should be followed by the application of a soothing antiseptic lotion that tingles but does not burn.

Step Six: Twin Masks

Two masks will then be applied, varying according to your skin type. The purpose of the masks is to complete the cleansing and soothing process, to help the skin recover and regain its "quiet."

The first mask will be a "tightening" mask containing natural deep sea mud, camphor or soothing antiseptic herbs. It will leave the skin feeling refreshed, stimulated, and pepped up.

The second mask is a more nourishing, soothing, moisturizing mask. It might be a honey and egg mixture or a fruit and vegetable mix blended with collagen or elastin moisturizers, depending on your skin's particular needs. Each mask will be left on for several minutes (not until it hardens but until it sets) and smoothly removed with cotton dipped in warm spring water. The neck and eye cream will be left on along with the mask, then cleaned off as well.

Finishing Touches

If this is your first facial and your skin is very dry and flaky, a light peeling mask may be applied to whisk away dry skin cells and surface flakiness. Every facial finishes with a spray of skin freshener and a light moisturizer plus a final application of eye cream.

Your skin should look radiant, glowing, refreshed—and your spirits should feel rejuvenated as well!

SKIN CARE NO-NOS

Always seek out a skin care expert who has experience with men's skin. Look for a specialist whose approach is informative, not pushy; you want information, not mere product sales talk. If you would feel uncomfortable going to a salon where most of the clients are women, then ask for the ratio of female to male clients when you call to make your appointment. One thing I cannot emphasize enough is the importance of personal rapport between you and the skin care salon staff. Look for someone who is honest with you, who does not overpromise/oversell/overexaggerate—if they do, they are likely to disappoint you. Nothing should be rushed. The atmosphere should be calming, peaceful.

Some signs that a skin care salon is less than expert; if the massage is done after the cleansing (this can aggravate skin oiliness and cause post-facial breakouts); if your skin is very red and blotchy when you leave the salon; if your skin feels irritated at any point during the facial. If you happen to have one bad experience with a salon, don't give up on skin care for good. As with any profession, there are the good and bad, the qualified and unqualified so-called experts.

Watch out for anyone who urges you to sign up for a series of treatments before you've even had one, or for anyone who urges you to buy a shopping bag full of products to use every day. While it is very true that the care you give your skin at home is very important to the outcome of any skin care, you do not need a complicated at-home routine. I always suggest to a man that he consider using one of my cleansing lotions and moisturizers appropriate to his skin type. If he enjoys it, he may want to "graduate" to a more involved skin care routine—or he may not. If a man tells me he wants to spend a maximum of two minutes a day on his skin, I'll help him make the most of those two minutes. Skin care should not be something that is imposed on you; it should be something you choose to spend time on. I urge clients to come back in a week or so (or call me) to let me know how the products are working, if they enjoy using them, if their skin seems to be reacting well. I feel it is my—and every skin care salon's—responsibility to offer to exchange or refund any product that a client does not like, or that does not react well with their skin. After all, my expertise and personal attention is what separates me from a cosmetics salesperson, and I want to know if anything goes wrong. My caring for the clients in my salon does not end when they walk out the door after a facial; it continues in the care I recommend at home. Never hesitate to let a skin care salon know of any complaints you have with their products. True experts will be glad to look into the problem, checking whether you are using the products correctly, as often as is needed, and whether you need a slight shift in product formula or type.

Don't feel that going to a skin specialist once means a lifelong commitment. Depending on your skin type, a salon may suggest an annual schedule of four facials, at the beginning of each switch of season, or they may suggest something more frequent. These are only suggestions, though; you must decide how much time you want to commit to regular skin care. A man can have beautiful skin and want to come every month for the relaxing benefits of the facial, or he may have very oily skin but have time for only three facials a year. The schedule you choose is up to you; beware of anyone who pushes you to choose one that is not suited to your lifestyle.

A skin care salon that promises instant results is a sham. Just as skin irritations or eruptions do not develop overnight, they cannot be cured in a single facial. Every skin is different and takes its own time in healing itself. You cannot have skin like your neighbor's, your friend's, or someone you saw in the movies last night—even if you all go to the same skin care specialist! Men are often impatient with skin care, but you must realize that it is a process that takes time. You will see improvement in your skin even after a single treatment, but it will not be a complete change. If you have neglected your skin for 30 years, you cannot expect a single visit to my salon—or to any other salon—to erase all of that damage! What I **can** do is to make your skin cleaner, smoother, and to help it look better and better as time goes on.

SKIN RENEWAL:
THE SALON PEEL—LIA'S WAY

Many men come to my salon with badly-scarred skin that has gotten over acne but still bears its aftereffects, or with very wrinkly, crepey skin that tells the tale of too many years of basking in the sun. In some cases, these men need more than a facial. What they need is a treatment that, six days later, can give them clearer, younger-looking skin. But I have just said that nothing works overnight, right? What I am talking about now is not merely a facial, but a skin makeover. It is a salon deep-peeling treatment, a mixture of vegetables, enzymes, herbs, and gentle chemicals that literally peels away the top four layers of skin and prods the body to produce new skin, pepping up a dull complexion, decreasing fine lines, and evening out some uneven pigmentation. What separates a salon peel from one done in a dermatologist's or plastic surgeon's office is the depth to which it peels the skin; a salon peel is kinder, safer on the skin, but it also cannot have the same depths of results as a surgical treatment.

This is not a treatment that is right for everyone. It cannot correct certain problems, and is best for **fine**—not deep—lines and scars. For example, a man came to my salon after visiting several other salons for consultations. He told me he wanted a salon peel. He had been told that he needed one by several other salons. I examined his skin under the magnifying lamp and saw that his acne scars were quite deep. I explained that a salon peel could not possibly erase such deep scars, but could only lessen them slightly. His skin would be somewhat smoother but would by no means be perfect after a salon peel. I also explained that he might want to talk to a physician about a dermabrasion treatment, as this goes deeper into the skin and erases deeper lines. He thanked me for my time and said he would go home and think about it, although he did not want to take the additional time off from work that a dermabrasion would require. Within a week, he was back in my salon and said that he had decided he wanted to go ahead with a salon peel in my salon because I had been so honest with him and he was willing to compromise in his expectations. This is a very important story, because unfortunately some salons will promise more than they can truly deliver—a fact that will only set a man up for disappointment later on. I did the salon peel on this man's skin, which looked better than even I had expected after the treatment, although it was still not perfect. Still, because the man knew what to expect, he was happy with the results.

One thing that is important to realize: With a salon peel you will have to take six days off from shaving, which for many men means six days off from work as well if your job requires a clean-shaven look.

The peeling mask must be applied once a day, left on for 1½ hours, then smoothed off. After each application, your skin will look red, as if you've been out in the sun. It will not be raw or blistery, like a surgical peel, nor will it be as painful. On the first few days, you may feel a slight burning sensation after the mask has been applied, but no more. While dermabrasion and physician peels take weeks to fully heal, with a salon peel, your skin returns to normal on day seven. Salon peeling can lessen acne scarring and curtail skin oiliness, and its benefits will last for up to a year.

A man of any age can benefit from a salon peel, although it should not be done on active acne breakouts. The only other contraindication is that you should not be taking antibiotics before or during the treatments. You should also not go out into the sun during the treatment, and should use a higher SPF sunscreen afterward, as your "newly born" skin will be more sun-sensitive. Your skin will look younger and more renewed, but the change won't be so drastic that anyone will know you've had a special treatment done. In fact, one client of mine who has a salon peel every other year often tells me that everyone comments on how wonderful he looks after his vacation—when he hasn't even left town!

AN AT-HOME FACIAL: LIA'S WAY

If you can't get to a skin care salon or want to boost the benefits, say, of three visits a year by giving your skin a facial at home once or twice, here is some safe advice for most skin types. (If you have acne or very dry or very sensitive skin, always go over these instructions with a skin care specialist before trying them at home to be sure to give your skin the best results possible.)

Part One: Cleansing

- Wash hands with soap and water.
- Apply liquid cleanser (or a creamy version) with a cotton ball, using gentle up-and-down motions on your face.
- Take another cotton ball, soaked in toning lotion, to complete the cleansing and to refresh your skin. Apply to face, using a gentle circular motion.

Part Two: Massage

- Take a tablespoonful of a rich, thick moisturizing cream in the palm of each hand. With palms only, massage your cheeks in a mild circular motion, moving from the center of the cheeks out toward the hairline. Do the same on your forehead. (If your skin tends to be oily, use a light moisturizer or a gel-formula moisturizer.)
- Use your index fingers to pat cream gently around the eyes, moving from the outer corners of the eyes inward toward the nose. Never rub or pull the skin.
- If you have dry skin, use index and middle fingers to massage cream onto your nose and chin. Omit this step if you have oily or combination skin.
- Massage cream into your neck, using a gentle up-and-down massage.

Part Three: Steam and Moisture

- Place chamomile leaves in a pot of just-boiled water. Improvise a towel tent over your head and steam your skin for three to five minutes.
- Cleanse off the moisturizer with cleansing lotion.
- Apply a nourishing mask appropriate to your skin type (either one prescribed for you by a skin care expert or one prepared from recipes earlier in this book).

● Leave mask on for 15 minutes; rinse off using lots of lukewarm water. Finish with a cool water splash. Apply a moisturizer appropriate to your skin type while skin is slightly damp to lock in moisture.

AT-HOME FACE MASSAGE: LIA'S WAY

While a facial massage can be relaxing and a good way to take your mind off the worries of the day, it is **not** a substitute for a face lift, nor can it truly change the muscles of the face. In fact, our facial muscles need no more "exercising" than they get in the course of every day. They are probably the most hard-working of our body's muscles, as we use them to smile, to talk, and to chew throughout every day of our lives. Some dermatologists caution that so-called facial exercises may actually do more harm than good, as wrinkling is in part caused by the continual movements of our facial tissues. A light massage can do no harm and is certainly relaxing. Don't press too hard—you want to soothe the face, not work it.

● Clean your face thoroughly before beginning, and wash your hands as well.

● Using the palms of your hands, gently stroke your forehead from one temple to another.

● Use the same movement from chin to temples.

● Stroke the corners of the jawbone, moving down to the neck and shoulders.

● Use the balls of your fingers to massage gently the tops of the cheeks, under, but not close to, the eyes. Start near the nose and work your way out to the edges of the face.

● Use the ends of your fingers to tap gently on the skin of the face. Start at the center of the forehead, moving out to the temples, and down along the edges of the face, ending at the center of the chin. Repeat, this time beginning at the cheeks and working down to the chin and increasing the tempo slightly. Repeat several times, increasing then decreasing the tempo, then slowing down to a stop.

MACHINES: DO THEY WORK?

Many professional facials include the use of Star Wars-inspired, futuristic-looking machinery, said to do everything from vacuuming dirt out of the pores to erasing wrinkles to lifting up nourishment from the lower levels of the skin to the top. In my 18 years of skin care experience, I have yet to see a machine that could truly meet any of these claims. Before founding my own salon, I worked at a famed New York City salon for two years that relied heavily on the use of such machines. Through using them myself, I am sorry to report, I saw firsthand how little they actually did—aside from increasing the cost of certain salon treatments.

The only machines you will find in my salon are a vaporizer-steam machine and an electric facial cleansing brush, which I use to thoroughly cleanse away skin flakiness on very dry skin. The vaporizer allows for more exact temperature control—and more safety—in steaming a client's face than does bending over a simple bowl of water. It also allows the client to relax more thoroughly by lying back in the chair during the steaming process than does sitting upright and bending over a bowl. The facial brush is excellent for removing excess skin flakiness from between the brows, along the edges of the nose and the chin—and is to be used only on certain skin types. A brush should never be used on highly sensitive skin or on acne breakouts; beware of a salon that uses the same equipment throughout every facial. Neither of the machines I use replaces any other steps of the facial, nor do they work miracles. They simply offer more efficiency in serving my client's needs.

Electrical stimulation of the face is often claimed to "cure" or "erase" wrinkles. If these machines don't work, you ask, why are they so often claimed to do so? Some dermatologists theorize that these machines **seem** to work because they subject the skin to micro-injuries. The skin's response to such injury is to summon increased fluid and injury-fighting white blood cells to the areas. This in turn results in a slight puffing up of the skin that masks any small wrinkles and thereby gives the illusion of having "erased" them. Within hours, unfortunately, when the swelling has subsided, the wrinkles have returned. The catch: when you leave the salon, you think that your wrinkles are gone!

In the long run, this repeated puffing up of the skin can stretch it out, eventually leading to more—not fewer—wrinkles. After all, no one has ever recommended sticking your finger into an electric socket to improve your health, so why should you subject your skin to repeated mini-electric shocks?

Be especially wary of any machinery used on the sensitive areas around the eyes or above the upper lip. These areas of the face have few if any oil glands and are very sensitive to injury and broken blood vessels. Using machines here could cause scarring later on.

In summary, while facial machinery may look modern and hi-tech, like the latest in scientific advances, it can actually cover up a practitioner's lack of skin knowledge. Anyone can buy a few machines and set himself up as a skin authority. But you are smart enough to know that a good skin care expert needs to know more than how to turn on a machine.

WHERE TO GO FOR THE BEST IN SKIN CARE ADVICE

In every city of the country—and in many a small town—skin care salons are opening faster than they can be counted. How do you judge the good from the bad? One way, as I have said before, is by increasing your own knowledge of sensible skin care, which has been the purpose of my writing—and your reading—this book. Another way is by going in for a consultation and assessing the advice you are given. Grooming or style editors of major magazines and newspapers are an often-overlooked source of referrals. They visit a wide variety of salons in their reporting and research, and it's their job to tell the good from the bad. They can often provide several reputable names in your area; how you evaluate their advice is up to you.

I would welcome any of my readers to visit my salon in New York City for a consultation if you live in or visit the area. As I could not, of course, treat all of my readers across the country, I offer this short list of other salons in major cities that have established reputations for being knowledgeable and for caring about their clients as individuals, which is, of course, an important factor in choosing a skin care salon:

NYC: LIA SCHORR
                686 Lexington Avenue
                4th Floor
                New York, NY 10022
                (212) 486-9670

CALIFORNIA: AIDA THIBIANT
                449 North Cannon Drive
                Beverly Hills, CA 90210
                (213) 278-7565

                LABELLE
                575 Sutter Street
                San Francisco, CA 94102
                (415) 433-7644

ARIZONA: Leah Kovitz
                NEW IMAGE
                8391 E. Hillwood Lane
                Tucson, AZ 85715
                (602) 298-5801

ILLINOIS: Leah Kovitz
                NEW IMAGE
                471 Lake Cook Road
                Deerfield, IL 60015
                (312) 564-8560

MASSACHUSETTS: ELIZABETH GRADY
181 Parking Way
Quincy, MA 02169
(617) 479-5800

TEXAS: GEORGETTE KLINGER
Dallas Parkway
Dallas, TX 75240
(214) 385-9393

LOUISIANA: LULU BURAS
Uras 2231 Banks Street
New Orleans, LA 70119
(504) 821-5144

FOR ADDITIONAL INFORMATION

To find out more about **electrolysis,** send a stamped, self-addressed envelope to:

THE INTERNATIONAL GUILD OF
PROFESSIONAL ELECTROLOGISTS
Medical Center
15 Bond Street
Great Neck, NY 11021

For more information on **dermatology,** or for a referral to a qualified dermatologist in your area, write to:

THE AMERICAN ACADEMY OF DERMATOLOGY
1567 Maple Avenue
Evanston, IL 60201

For information on specific **plastic surgery** procedures, or to be referred to a qualified surgeon in your area, write to:

THE AMERICAN SOCIETY OF PLASTIC
AND RECONSTRUCTIVE SURGEONS
233 North Michigan Avenue
Chicago, IL 60611

To get help with a **drinking problem,** look under "alcoholism" in your local phone book. There you'll find listings for the local branch of Alcoholics Anonymous as well as Alanon, the support groups for families of those with drinking problems. You'll also find listings for support groups at local medical centers and area hospitals. You can also find local public health programs listed in the "government office" section of your city phone book.

To get help with a **drug problem,** contact your local hospital or look under "drug abuse" in your local phone book. Your local physician can also refer you to groups in your area, as can church or synagogue personnel, school district personnel, and many corporate health service programs, more and more of which are recognizing the need for support for employees who develop drug problems.

INDEX